World Review of Nutrition and Dietetics

Vol. 109

Series Editor

Berthold Koletzko Munich

Nutrition and Growth
Yearbook 2014

Volume Editors

Berthold Koletzko Munich

Raanan Shamir Petach-Tikva/Tel Aviv

Dominique Turck Lille

Moshe Phillip Petach-Tikva/Tel Aviv

2014

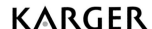

KARGER Basel · Freiburg · Paris · London · New York · Chennai · New Delhi · Bangkok · Beijing · Shanghai · Tokyo · Kuala Lumpur · Singapore · Sydney

Berthold Koletzko
Div. Metabolic and Nutritional Medicine
Dr. von Hauner Children's Hospital
Univ. of Munich Medical Centre –
Klinikum d. Univ. München
München
Germany

Dominique Turck
Division of Gastroenterology
Hepatology and Nutrition
Department of Pediatrics
Jeanne de Flandre Children's Hospital
And Lille University Faculty of Medicine
INSERM U995
Lille
France

Raanan Shamir
Institute of Gastroenterology
Nutrition and Liver Diseases
Schneider Children's Medical Center of Israel
Clalit Health Services
Petach-Tikva, Israel
And Sackler School of Medicine
Tel Aviv University
Tel Aviv
Israel

Moshe Phillip
Jesse Z and Sara Lea Shafer Institute for
Endocrinology and Diabetes
National Center for Childhood Diabetes
Schneider Children's Medical Center of Israel
Petach-Tikva
And Sackler Faculty of Medicine
Tel Aviv University
Tel Aviv
Israel

Library of Congress Cataloging-in-Publication Data

Nutrition and growth (Koletzko)
  Nutrition and growth : yearbook 2014 / volume editors, Berthold Koletzko,
Raanan Shamir, Dominique Turck, Moshe Phillip.
     p. ; cm. -- (World review of nutrition and dietetics, ISSN 0084-2230
; vol. 109)
  Includes bibliographical references and indexes.
  ISBN 978-3-318-02565-1 (hbk. : alk. paper) -- ISBN 978-3-318-02566-8
(electronic version)
  I. Koletzko, B. (Berthold), editor of compilation. II. Shamir, Raanan,
editor of compilation. III. Turck, Dominique, editor of compilation. IV.
Phillip, Moshe, editor of compilation. V. Title. VI. Series: World review of
nutrition and dietetics ; v. 109. 0084-2230
  [DNLM: 1. Growth and Development--physiology--Collected Works. 2. Child
Nutritional Physiological Phenomena--Collected Works. 3. Maternal
Nutritional Physiological Phenomena--Collected Works. W1 WO898 v.109 2014 /
WS 103]
  QP84
  612.6--dc23
                                            2013044986

Bibliographic Indices. This publication is listed in bibliographic services, including Current Contents® and PubMed/MEDLINE.

Disclaimer. The statements, opinions and data contained in this publication are solely those of the individual authors and contributors and not of the publisher and the editor(s). The appearance of advertisements in the book is not a warranty, endorsement, or approval of the products or services advertised or of their effectiveness, quality or safety. The publisher and the editor(s) disclaim responsibility for any injury to persons or property resulting from any ideas, methods, instructions or products referred to in the content or advertisements.

Drug Dosage. The authors and the publisher have exerted every effort to ensure that drug selection and dosage set forth in this text are in accord with current recommendations and practice at the time of publication. However, in view of ongoing research, changes in government regulations, and the constant flow of information relating to drug therapy and drug reactions, the reader is urged to check the package insert for each drug for any change in indications and dosage and for added warnings and precautions. This is particularly important when the recommended agent is a new and/or infrequently employed drug.

© Copyright 2014 by S. Karger AG, P.O. Box, CH–4009 Basel (Switzerland)
www.karger.com
Printed in Germany on acid-free and non-aging paper (ISO 9706) by Kraft Druck, Ettlingen
ISSN 0084–2230
e-ISSN 1662–3975
ISBN 978–3–318–02565–1
e-ISBN 978–3–318–02566–8

Contents

List of Contributors

S. Faisal Ahmed
Developmental Endocrinology Research Group
Royal Hospital for Sick Children
University of Glasgow
Yorkhill
Glasgow G3 8SJ (UK)
E-Mail: Faisal.Ahmed@glasgow.ac.uk

Mabrouka A. Altowati
Developmental Endocrinology Research Group
Royal Hospital for Sick Children
University of Glasgow
Yorkhill
Glasgow G3 8SJ (UK)
E-Mail: m.altowati.1@research.gla.ac.uk

Jeffrey Baron
National Institute of Child Health and
Human Development
National Institutes of Health, CRC, Room 1-3330
10 Center Drive, MSC-1103
Bethesda, MD 20892-1103 (USA)
E-Mail: baronj@cc1.nichd.nih.gov

Tadej Battelino
Department of Pediatric Endocrinology
Diabetes and Metabolism
UMC-University Children's Hospital
Bohoriceva 20
SLO-1000 Ljubljana (Slovenia)
E-Mail: tadej.battelino@mf.uni-lj.si

Zulfiqar A. Bhutta
Aga Khan University Hospital, Karachi
Stadium Road, PO Box 3500
PK-74800 Karachi (Pakistan)
E-Mail: zulfiqar.bhutta@aku.edu

Susan E. Carlson
University of Kansas Medical Center
Department of Dietetics and Nutrition
MS 4013, 3901 Rainbow Boulevard
Kansas City, KS 66160 (USA)
E-Mail: scarlson@kumc.edu

Corina Hartmen
Institute of Gastroenterology
Nutrition and Liver Diseases
Schneider Children's Medical Center of Israel
Clalit Health Services
Petach-Tikva, Israel
And Sackler School of Medicine
Tel Aviv University
IL-39040 Tel Aviv (Israel)
E-Mail: CorinaH@clalit.org.il

Liran Hiersch
Helen Schneider Hospital for Women
Rabin Medical Center
Petach-Tikva, Israel
And the Sackler Faculty of Medicine
Tel Aviv University
IL-39040 Tel Aviv (Israel)
E-Mail: liranH@clalit.org.il

Holly R. Hull
University of Kansas Medical Center
Department of Dietetics and Nutrition
MS 4013, 3901 Rainbow Boulevard
Kansas City, KS 66160 (USA)
E-Mail: hhull@kumc.edu

Youn Hee Jee
National Institute of Child Health and
Human Development
National Institutes of Health, CRC
Room 1-3330
10 Center Drive, MSC-1103
Bethesda, MD 20892-1103 (USA)
E-Mail: youn.jee@nih.gov

Berthold Koletzko
Division of Metabolic and Nutritional Medicine
Dr. von Hauner Children's Hospital
University of Munich Medical Centre
Lindwurmstr. 4
DE-80337 Munich (Germany)
E-Mail: Office.Koletzko@med.uni-muenchen.de

Luis A. Moreno
GENUD (Growth, Exercise, NUtrition and
Development) Research Group
Department of Physiatry and Nursing
Faculty of Health Sciences
C/Domingo Miral s/n
ES-50009 Zaragoza (Spain)
E-Mail: lmoreno@unizar.es

Moshe Phillip
The Jesse Z and Sara Lea Shafer Institute for
Endocrinology and Diabetes
National Center for Childhood Diabetes
Schneider Children's Medical Center of Israel
14 Kaplan Street
IL-4920235 Petach-Tikva (Israel)
E-Mail: mosheph@post.tau.ac.il

Raanan Shamir
Institute of Gastroenterology
Nutrition and Liver Diseases
Schneider Children's Medical Center of Israel
Professor of Pediatrics, Sackler Faculty of
Medicine, Tel Aviv University
14 Kaplan St.
IL-49202 Petach-Tikva (Israel)
E-Mail: RaananS@clalit.org.il

J.B. Hans van Goudoever
Academic Medical Center
University of Amsterdam
Meibergdreef 9
NL-1105 AZ Amsterdam (The Netherlands)
E-Mail: h.vangoudoever@amc.uva.nl

Dominique Turck
Division of Gastroenterology
Hepatology and Nutrition
Department of Pediatrics
Jeanne de Flandre Children's Hospital
Lille University Faculty of Medicine
INSERM U995
Avenue Eugène Avinée
FR-59037 Lille cedex (France)
E-Mail: DTURCK@CHRU-LILLE.FR

Yariv Yogev
Helen Schneider Hospital for Women
Rabin Medical Center
Petach-Tikva, Israel
And the Sackler Faculty of Medicine
Tel Aviv University
IL-39040 Tel Aviv (Israel)
E-Mail: yarivy@clalit.org.il

Preface

The relation between nutrition and growth in children is one of the key concerns of child health. The interaction between nutrition and growth poses a challenge to pediatricians, including subspecialists in pediatric nutrition, endocrinology and gastroenterology, pediatric nutritionists and dieticians, and other health professionals involved in the care of children. Thus, exchanging concepts and knowledge between the professionals of all the different disciplines is key to facilitating research and interdisciplinary clinical collaborations.

The growing interest in the relationship between nutrition and growth gave rise to numerous articles in various medical journals. With this in mind, we decided on publishing the first *Yearbook on Nutrition and Growth*. The main idea is to bring to practicing physicians succinct editorial comments, evaluating the clinical importance of each article and to discuss its application. The articles discussed in this book are those that have the most important potential contribution in the field. The studies might contribute to a better understanding of the mechanism of interactions, the way of thinking, the existing concepts in the field or that may lead to a change in the way we treat our patients.

The editors of the different chapters of the *Yearbook* are renowned experts in their fields who kindly agreed to share their views and wisdom. This first *Yearbook on Nutrition and Growth* is based on articles published from 1 July 2012 to 30 June 2013. We hope you will find the book useful for your work.

Berthold Koletzko, Munich
Raanan Shamir, Petach-Tikva/Tel Aviv
Dominique Turck, Lille
Moshe Phillip, Petach-Tikva/Tel Aviv

Koletzko B, Shamir R, Turck D, Phillip M (eds): Nutrition and Growth: Yearbook 2014.
World Rev Nutr Diet. Basel, Karger, 2014, vol 109, pp 1–22 (DOI: 10.1159/000356352)

Obesity, Metabolic Syndrome and Nutrition

Tadej Battelino[1] and Shlomit Shalitin[2]

[1] UMC-University Children's Hospital and Faculty of Medicine, University of Ljubljana, Ljubljana, Slovenia
[2] The Jesse Z. and Sara Lea Shafer Institute of Endocrinology & Diabetes National Center for Childhood Diabetes Schneider Children's Medical Center of Israel, Petach-Tikva and Sackler Faculty of Medicine, Tel Aviv University, Tel Aviv, Israel

Over the span of the last decades there has been an alarming worldwide increase in childhood obesity [1], which tends to track into adulthood [2]. Childhood obesity is associated with a significant risk for the development of type 2 diabetes, hypertension, dyslipidemia, metabolic syndrome, and is also a risk factor for early cardiovascular events. The timing of the obesity epidemic is parallel to the increased availability of calorie-dense foods and a more sedentary lifestyle – the 'obesogenic environment' [3]. However, not all individuals become obese while living in the same environment. Therefore, variability among individuals is suspected to result from heritability of obesity susceptibility genes that interact with components in the 'obesogenic environment' to promote positive energy balance responsible for weight gain [4].

Recent evidence, primarily from animal studies and observational data in humans, suggests that the epigenome can be altered by maternal diet during the periconceptional period and that these programming events may underlie later disease risk. In one of the works cited below it was demonstrated that the periconceptual micronutrients altered methylation at the differentially methylated regions of imprinted genes associated with obesity. These results may support the concept that nutrition in critical periods of life can permanently influence the development of chronic diseases. The 'obesogenic environment' is a complex of contributing factors that influence the dietary choice, physical activity, or metabolism responsible for maintaining energy balance. Both sedentary behavior and reduced physical activity promote the overconsumption of dietary macronutrients, particularly fats and refined carbohydrates [5].

It is widely accepted that high-fat diets, characterized by enhanced palatability and high-energy density, may be primarily responsible for the current obesity epidemic. Also, increased consumption of carbohydrates, particularly refined carbohydrates and sugar-sweetened beverages, can contribute to the increased prevalence of obesity [6]. The dietary pattern, food frequency, and breakfast consumption may also have an impact on body weight and on markers of the metabolic syndrome. Finally, the connection between gut microbiota, energy homeostasis, and inflammation and its role in the pathogenesis of obesity-related disorders are emerging as a new break for intervention. Although current childhood obesity intervention programs have traditionally focused only on generalized population guidelines, further investigation and insight into gene-diet interactions may serve an important role in both the prevention and treatment of childhood obesity by using targeted nutritional and drug therapies. This chapter reviews a selection of important articles published between July 2012 and June 2013 focusing on the relation between nutrition, obesity and metabolic syndrome in the pediatric age group.

DNA methylation profiling at imprinted loci after periconceptional micronutrient supplementation in humans: results of a pilot randomized controlled trials

Cooper WN[1], Khulan B[1,2], Owens S[5], Elks CE[6], Seidel V[1], Prentice AM[5], Belteki G[3,7], Ong KK[3,4], Affara NA[2], Constância M[1,4,8], Dunger DB[3,8]

[1]Metabolic Research Laboratories, Department of Obstetrics and Gynaecology, [2]Department of Pathology, [3]Department of Paediatrics, and [4]Centre for Trophoblast Research, University of Cambridge, Cambridge, UK; [5]Medical Research Council (MRC) International Nutrition Group, London School of Hygiene and Tropical Medicine, London, UK; [6]MRC Epidemiology Unit, Institute of Metabolic Science, Cambridge, UK; [7]Neonatal Intensive Care Unit, Cambridge University Hospitals NHS Foundation Trust, Rosie Hospital, Cambridge, UK; [8]National Institute for Health Research, Cambridge Biomedical Research Centre, Cambridge, UK

FASEB J 2012; 26: 1782–1790

Background: Nutrition around conception and during pregnancy was associated with earlier onset of diseases of affluence, particularly coronary heart disease (CHD), obesity and type 2 diabetes (T2D). Several animal trials support these observations, however no randomized controlled trial existed to test this in humans. The influence of nutrition on epigenome (DNA methylation and histone modification) could at least in part cause the observed association. Imprinted genes confer monoallelic (from 1 parent) expression of one or more transcripts likely to be caused by different methylation of differentially methylated regions (DMRs). The methylation imprints at maternally methylated gametic DMRs are thought to be set up postnatally during the final stages of oocyte maturation and may be particularly susceptible to nutritional insufficiencies in the pre- and periconceptional period. After fertilization, methylation at gametic DMRs resists genome-wide demethylation events that occur in early embryo until implantation.

Aims: The randomized controlled trial of United Nations International Multiple Micronutrient Preparation (UNIMMAP) periconceptional supplementation in rural Gambia was utilized to investigate if periconceptional nutritional exposures affect DNA methylation at imprinted loci.

Methods: Non-pregnant women aged 17–45 were randomized to receive daily supplementation with either UNIMMAP or placebo. Once pregnancy was confirmed in a woman who ceased supplementation. DNA was extracted from cord blood of 22 newborns of compliant mothers in the intervention group and 36 newborns from the control group. The loci chosen for quantification of methylation using mass spectrometry included paternally or maternally methylated germline and somatic DMRs, previously associated with known human disorders (Prader-Willi syndrome, Angelman syndrome, Beckwith-Wiedemann syndrome, Silver-Russell syndrome, pseudohypoparathyroidism, and transient neonatal diabetes mellitus syndrome).

Results: The difference in methylation was statistically significant for 2 of the 13 regions, IGF2R-DMR and GTL2-DMR_2, when analyzed separately by gender. UNIMMAP intervention significantly reduced methylation levels at IGF2R-DMR in girls and GTL2-DMR_2 in boys.

Conclusions: Despite several limitations of this trial the present observations indicate that from a randomized controlled trial independent of seasonal effects, periconceptional nutrition could influence gender-specific methylation of critical fetal imprints.

Comments   This study provides preliminary pilot results obtained in nucleated cells from cord blood. The statistical analysis did not include Bonferroni correction for multiple comparisons and thus the results may not be statistically significant using a more rigorous analysis. Additionally, findings from the cord blood were not confirmed in samples taken at the age of 9 months. Despite several important limitations, this is the first randomized controlled trial demonstrating that periconceptual micronutrients may alter methylation at the DMRs in imprinted genes. If confirmed in a larger trial, these results may support an important concept that nutrition in critical periods of life can permanently influence the development of chronic diseases.

Sexual dimorphism in the early life programming of serum leptin levels in European adolescents: the HELENA study

Labayen I[1,2], Ruiz JR[3,4], Huybrechts I[5], Ortega FB[6], Rodríguez G[2], Dehenauw S[5], Breidenassel C[7], Jiménez-Pavón D[6], Vyncke KE[5], Censi L[8], Molnar D[9], Widhalm K[10], Kafatos A[11], Plada M[11], Díaz LE[12], Marcos A[12], Moreno LA[2], Gottrand F[13,14]

[1]Department of Nutrition and Food Science, University of the Basque Country, Vitoria, Spain; [2]GENUD (Growth, Exercise, Nutrition, and Development) Research Group, Faculty of Medicine and Department of Pediatrics, Instituto Aragonés de Ciencias de la Salud, and University School of Health Sciences, University of Zaragoza, Zaragoza, Spain; [3]Department of Physical Education, School of Physical Education and Sport Sciences, University of Granada, Granada, Spain; [4]Unit for Preventive Nutrition, Department of Biosciences and Nutrition at NOVUM, Karolinska Institutet, Huddinge, Sweden; [5]Department of Public Health, Faculty of Medicine, Ghent University, and Department of Nutrition and Dietetics, Faculty of Health Care Vesalius, University College Ghent, Belgium; [6]Department of Medical Physiology, School of Medicine, University of Granada, Spain; [7]Department of Nutrition and Food Science, University of Bonn, Germany; [8]National Research Institute on Food and Nutrition, Rome, Italy; [9]Department of Pediatrics, University of Pecs, Pecs, Hungary; [10]Division of Nutrition and Metabolism, Department of Pediatrics, Medical University of Vienna, Vienna, Austria; [11]University of Crete School of Medicine, Crete, Greece; [12]Immunonutrition Research Group, Department of Metabolism and Nutrition, Spanish Council for Scientific Research, Madrid, Spain; [13]Institut National de la Santé et de la Recherche Médicale Unité 995, IFR 114, Faculty of Medicine, University of Lille 2, Lille, France; [14]Department of Pediatrics, Jeanne de Flandre Children's University Hospital, Lille, France

J Clin Endocrinol Metab 2011; 96: E1330–E1334

Background: Adverse intrauterine circumstances reflected in lower birth weight are associated with earlier onset of chronic diseases such as obesity and type 2 diabetes.

Aims: This study tested the relationship between birth weight and serum leptin concentration in adolescents, and its possible gender dimorphism.

Methods: Healthy Lifestyle in Europe by Nutrition in Adolescence (HELENA) cross-sectional study involved 3,546 adolescents. The present study selected 757 adolescents born at >37 weeks after amenorrhea with complete and valid data on birth weight, serum leptin concentration, body mass index (BMI), and pubertal status (Tanner). Physical activity was assessed with accelerometry over 7 days. Fasting serum leptin concentrations were measured with ELISA.

Results: There was a significant interaction between birth weight and gender on serum leptin levels ($p < 0.04$). Body weight at birth was significantly negatively associated with serum leptin levels in female adolescents controlled for center, duration of gestation and breastfeeding, pubertal status, and BMI. Results remained significant when controlled for physical activity ($\beta = -0.115$; $p = 0.016$). Likewise, the results did not substantially change when the analysis was controlled for z-score BMI ($\beta -0.119$; $p = 0.003$), body fat percentage ($\beta = -0.100$; $p < 0.015$), or waist circumference ($\beta = -0.117$; $p = 0.006$) instead of BMI. Similarly, results remain significant when overweight and obese were excluded from the analysis.

Conclusions: Further evidence for a possible gender-specific programming effect of birth weight on the energy homeostasis in adolescence is provided. The association between lower birth weight and the increased long-term risk of developing obesity and type 2 diabetes may be in part mediated by different programming of energy metabolism.

Comments   This study has several limitations due to its retrospective (questionnaire-based) and cross-sectional design. Additionally, estrogen concentrations, known to influence leptin concentration in females, were not measured. However, reported results are in line with more than a few similar reports from animal models and are of obvious clinical relevance. Further prospective studies are warranted to investigate the relationship between intrauterine nutritional environment and later abundance-associated morbidity.

A trial of sugar-free or sugar-sweetened beverages and body weight in children

De Ruyter JC, Olthof MR, Seidell JC, Katan MB

Department of Health Sciences, EMGO Institute for Health and Care Research, VU University Amsterdam, Amsterdam, The Netherlands

N Engl J Med 2012; 367: 1397–1406

Background: Beverages containing sugar are assumed to cause a more significant increase in body weight than solid foods because they do not lead to a sense of satiety. Consumption of sugar-sweetened beverages may be associated with undiminished intake of calories from other foods and beverages, resulting in weight gain.

Aims: As the existing results were not conclusive, a Double-blind, Randomized Intervention Study in Kids (DRINK) was commenced to examine the effect of masked replacement of sugar-sweetened beverages with non-caloric, artificially sweetened beverages on weight gain.

Methods: In this 18-month, double-blind, randomized, controlled trial, 641 schoolchildren living in the community who were 4 years 10 months to 11 years 11 months of age were enrolled, stratified according to school, sex, age, and initial body mass index (BMI), and individually randomly assigned to 1 can daily of a non-caloric, artificially sweetened, non-carbonated beverage or a sugar-containing non-carbonated beverage. Children in the same household received the same type of blinded beverage. Body weight, height, skinfold thickness, waist circumference, and arm-to-leg electrical impedance were measured and urine samples at 0, 6, 12, and 18 months were collected. Adherence to the protocol was monitored.

Results: The adherence beverage consumption was 88% at 6 months, 81% at 12 months, and 74% at 18 months. Children who dropped out had a slightly higher BMI at baseline, and their parents had completed fewer years of school. The 477 children who completed the study consumed 5.8 out of 7 (83%) cans per week, with no difference between the groups or over time. The level of urinary sucralose confirmed the adherence in the control group. In the full cohort of 641 children with missing values imputed, the mean BMI z-score increased by 0.02 ± 0.41 SD units in the sugar-free group and by 0.15 ± 0.42 SD units in the sugar group; the mean difference of 0.13 SD units was significant, also when adjusted for age. The sugar-free group gained significantly less body fat, as evidenced by skinfold thickness, waist-to-height ratio, and electrical impedance. The mean weight increased by 6.35 ± 3.07 kg in the sugar-free group and by 7.37 ± 3.35 kg in the sugar group, with the mean difference of 1.01 kg being significant, also when adjusted for height change. Children in the sugar-free group who completed the study gained 35% less fat according to impedance measurements and 19% less fat according to four skinfolds measurements (a gain of 1.47 vs. 1.82 kg of body fat).

Conclusions: Weight gain and body fat gain in healthy children were significantly reduced by masked replacement of a sugar-containing beverage with a sugar-free beverage.

Comments   This study provides extremely important and strong evidence that sugar-sweetened beverages increase body weight and body fat in children. Similar results were obtained in adolescents, which considerably adds to the weight of evidence. Interestingly, further evidence suggests that sugar-sweetened beverages can have a particularly strong negative effect on persons genetically susceptible for obesity [7]. Taking this together, all professionals involved in the care of children and adolescents as well as parents and society as such should act upon this evidence and reduce the risks these young people are exposed to through sugar-sweetened beverages.

A randomized trial of sugar-sweetened beverages and adolescent body weight

Ebbeling CB[1], Feldman HA[2], Chomitz VR[3], Antonelli TA[2], Gortmaker SL[4], Osganian SK[2], Ludwig DS[1]

[1]The New Balance Foundation Obesity Prevention Center, Boston, MA, USA; [2]Clinical Research Center, Boston Children's Hospital, Boston, MA, USA; [3]Institute for Community Health, Cambridge, MA, USA; [4]Department of Society, Human Development, and Health, Harvard School of Public Health, Boston, MA, USA

N Engl J Med 2012; 367: 1407–1416

Background: The consumption of sugar-sweetened beverages among adolescents has increased in tandem with the prevalence of pediatric obesity, suggesting a causal relationship. At present, a substantial proportion of high-school students habitually consume sugar-sweetened beverages, including carbonated soda, energy drinks, and highly sweetened coffees and teas. Short-term feeding studies show greater energy intake and weight gain with the consumption of sugar-sweetened beverages than with beverages containing artificial sweeteners.

Objective: This study was designed to test the hypothesis that overweight and obese adolescents who received an intervention to reduce the consumption of sugar-sweetened beverages would gain weight at a slower rate than those who did not receive the intervention.

Methods: Overweight and obese adolescents who regularly consumed sugar-sweetened beverages (n = 224) were randomly assigned to intervention and control groups. The intervention group received a 1-year intervention designed to decrease consumption of sugar-sweetened beverages, with follow-up for an additional year without intervention.

Results: The retention rate for study participants was 97% at 1 year and 93% at 2 years, with no significant difference between groups in the percentage of participants available at 2 years for assessment of the primary outcome. Reported consumption of sugar-sweetened beverages was similar at baseline in the intervention and control groups (1.7 servings/day), declined to nearly zero in the intervention group at 1 year, and remained lower than in the control group at 2 years. The change in mean BMI at 2 years did not differ significantly between the groups. At 1 year, there were significant between-group differences for changes in BMI and weight. Only among Hispanic participants (27 in the intervention group, 19 in the control group) there was a significant between-group difference in the change in BMI at 1 and 2 years. The change in the percentage of body fat did not differ significantly between groups at 2 years.

Conclusions: The provision of non-caloric beverages virtually eliminated reported consumption of sugar-sweetened beverages and reduced total reported energy intake among overweight and obese adolescents after a 1-year intervention, with persistent effects on diet through follow-up at 2 years. Replacement of sugar-sweetened beverages with non-caloric beverages did not improve body weight over a 2-year period, but group differences in dietary quality and body weight were observed at the end of the 1-year intervention period.

Comments Over the past years, the notion of the coincident increase in sugar-sweetened beverages consumption with increased prevalence of obesity raised the possibility to limit the consumption of caloric soft drinks, especially in children and adolescents, in order to fight the epidemic of obesity. Caloric drinks are marketed for young people by intensive advertising strategies. These drinks may drive greater energy intake and weight gain through satiety signaling and compensatory dietary responses. A recent published paper [7] provides evidence that individuals with a more pronounced genetic predisposition to obesity may be more susceptible to the adverse effects of sugar-sweetened beverages on BMI. In the present study, education and behavioral counseling focused specifically on decreasing consumption of sugar-sweetened beverages, a single dietary behavior that may be particularly important for controlling body weight. The significant intervention effect for the change in BMI observed at 1 year, together with the findings of de Ruyter et al. (in the previous abstract), provides support for public health guidelines that recommend limiting consumption of sugar-sweetened beverages. The lack of effect at 2 years could reflect increasing energy intake from sugar-sweetened beverages or fruit juices in the intervention group on discontinuation of the intervention or decreasing intake of sugar-sweetened beverages or fruit juices in the control group, possibly due to the efforts to eliminate these beverages from schools.

Prospective associations between sugar-sweetened beverage intakes and cardiometabolic risk factors in adolescents

Ambrosini GL[1], Oddy WH [2], Huang RC[3,4], Mori TA[3], Beilin LJ[3], Jebb SA[1]

[1]The Medical Research Council Human Nutrition Research, Elsie Widdowson Laboratory, Cambridge, UK; [2]Telethon Institute for Child Health Research, Centre for Child Health Research, Perth, WA, Australia; [3]School of Medicine and Pharmacology, Royal Perth Hospital Unit, Perth, WA, Australia; [4]School of Paediatrics and Child Health, University of Western Australia, Perth, WA, Australia

Am J Clin Nutr 2013; 98: 327–334

Background: Sugar-sweetened beverages have been linked with weight gain, type 2 diabetes, and increased cardiovascular disease risk in adults. However, a better understanding of the relations between sugar-sweetened beverages and cardiometabolic health in children and adolescents is required. It was hypothesized that increases in sugar-sweetened beverages consumption between 14 and 17 years of age would be positively associated with a greater odds of overweight or obesity and unfavorable changes in cardiovascular disease risk factors, independent of body weight.

Objective: This study investigated prospective associations between sugar-sweetened beverages consumption and cardiometabolic risk factors in a cohort of adolescents for whom diet has been well characterized.

Methods: Data were provided by adolescents (n = 1,433) offspring from the Western Australian Pregnancy Cohort (Raine) Study, in which 2,900 pregnant women at 16–20 weeks' gestation were recruited through public and private antenatal clinics in Western Australia between 1989 and 1991. Of these subjects, 2,804 women (97%) had 2,868 live births. These children and their families have been followed up at regular intervals since. The data were derived from follow-ups at 14 and 17 years of age about sugar-sweetened beverages intakes estimated by a food-frequency questionnaire, and measurements of BMI, waist circumference (WC), blood pressure (BP), fasting serum lipids, glucose, and insulin. The overall cardiometabolic risk was estimated. Associations between sugar-sweetened beverages intake and cardiovascular disease risk factors were done adjusted for age, pubertal stage, physical fitness, socioeconomic status, and major dietary patterns.

Results: Sugar-sweetened beverages were the most consumed beverage type in both genders, and 89% of respondents were sugar-sweetened beverages consumers at each follow-up. Sugar-sweetened beverages provided 4–5% of total energy intakes of which ~50% came from carbonated or soft drinks. At baseline (14 years of age), the average BMI, WC, total energy intake, systolic BP, fasting triglycerides, and z-score for the Western dietary pattern increased, whereas the average HDL cholesterol, glucose, and z-score for the healthy dietary pattern decreased, with increasing intakes of sugar-sweetened beverages (p trend <0.05). The prevalence of obesity, low maternal education, and low family income increased with higher sugar-sweetened beverages intakes (p < 0.05). Girls who moved into the highest tertile of sugar-sweetened beverages consumption (>1.3 servings/day) between the ages 14 and 17 years had a 4.8 times greater odds of overweight or obesity (p trend <0.0001) and a 3 times greater odds (p trend = 0.001) of being classified at a greater metabolic risk at 17 years than did girls who remained in the lowest sugar-sweetened beverages tertile. These associations were not observed in boys. Compared with staying in the lowest sugar-sweetened beverages tertile, moving into the highest tertile of sugar-sweetened beverages intake between the ages 14 and 17 years was associated with an average increases in BMI of 3.8% (p trend <0.001) in girls, and with increases in WC in both genders. With higher sugar-sweetened beverages intakes, there was an increasing trend in fasting triglycerides in both genders (p trend ≤0.003), and decreasing in HDL cholesterol concentrations in boys (p trend ≤0.02), even after adjustment for total energy intake.

Conclusion: Greater sugar-sweetened beverages intakes during adolescence were prospectively associated with greater overweight and obesity risk and higher overall cardiometabolic risk in girls and unfavorable changes in WC and triglycerides (for both genders), and HDL cholesterol (for boys), independent of BMI.

Comments   Sugar-sweetened beverages which include carbonated (soft) drinks and fruit drinks with added sugar are supposed to increase obesity risk primarily because they provide a liquid form of energy that has less impact on satiety than isoenergetic food. Sugar-sweetened beverages may also have direct effects on cardiometabolic health, independent of weight gain. Experimental and observational studies have shown that high sugar-sweetened beverages consumption increases the dietary glycemic load, which can lead to insulin resistance, impaired β-cell function, and inflammation. In addition, high intakes of fructose sweeteners in sugar-sweetened beverages have been linked to visceral adiposity, hepatic lipogenesis, and hypertension [8]. The follow-up period in this cohort of adolescents was relatively short (2 years), and these changes may accumulate over time. Thus, the results of this study suggest that sugar-sweetened beverages consumption should be limited in young people not only for obesity prevention, but also in order to reduce future cardiometabolic risk.

Dietary salt intake, sugar-sweetened beverage consumption, and obesity risk

Grimes CA, Riddell LJ, Campbell KJ, Nowson CA

Centre for Physical Activity and Nutrition Research, School of Exercise and Nutrition Sciences, Deakin University, Burwood, VIC, Australia

Pediatrics 2013; 131: 14–21

Background: Greater consumption of sugar-sweetened beverages over the previous two decades may be associated with the rise in childhood obesity rates. Emerging evidence suggests that a reduction in dietary salt intake may reduce sugar-sweetened beverages consumption. The mechanism behind this relationship lies in the homeostatic trigger of thirst in response to the ingestion of dietary salt. It is suggested that in an environment where soft drinks are readily available, a high-salt diet may encourage greater consumption of soft drinks in children.
Objective: The aim was to examine the association between dietary salt intake, overall fluid consumption, as well as sugar-sweetened beverages consumption, and to examine the association between sugar-sweetened beverages consumption and weight status.
Methods: The study was based on cross-sectional data from the 2007 Australian National Children's Nutrition and Physical Activity Survey of children aged 2–16 years. Consumption of dietary salt, fluid, and sugar-sweetened beverages was determined via two 24-hour dietary recalls. Height and weight were recorded and served for BMI calculation. The association between salt, fluid, sugar-sweetened beverages consumption, and weight status was assessed using regression analysis.
Results: 62% of all the 4,283 participants reported consuming sugar-sweetened beverages, without a difference between genders. Salt intake and fluid consumption increased with age, with a positive correlation between salt intake and total fluid consumption ($r = 0.42$, $p < 0.001$), even after adjustment for age, gender, socioeconomic status (SES), and BMI ($p < 0.001$). Older age and lower SES were both significantly associated with higher sugar-sweetened beverages consumption (both $p < 0.001$). Consumers of sugar-sweetened beverages were more likely to be overweight and obese than non-consumers ($p < 0.05$). In sugar-sweetened beverages consumers (n = 2,571), salt intake was

positively associated with sugar-sweetened beverages consumption (r = 0.35, p < 0.001), adjusted for age, gender, SES, and energy (p < 0.001). Children who consumed >1 serving of sugar-sweetened beverages were 26% more likely to be overweight/obese (p < 0.01).

Conclusions: The consumption of sugar-sweetened beverages is relatively common in Australian children aged 2–16 years and dietary salt intake was positively associated with overall fluid consumption. Furthermore, within consumers of sugar-sweetened beverages, dietary salt intake predicted sugar-sweetened beverages consumption, which was associated with an increased risk of obesity.

Comments   The major strengths of this study include the use of a large, nationally representative sample of Australian children, with a comprehensive and standardized collection of dietary intake, anthropometric, and demographic data. Over the life course, minor changes in energy balance can increase the risk of obesity. In children on relatively high salt intakes, experiencing a drive for fluid, with easy access to sugar-sweetened beverages, a greater consumption of sugar-sweetened beverages may occur. The consumption of sugar-sweetened soft drinks is associated with reduced vegetable and milk consumption (typically low-salt foods) and higher consumption of fast food (e.g. hamburgers and french fries, typically high-salt foods). Thus, it is possible that some of the association reported in the current study is a result of the overall clustering of 'unhealthy' dietary behaviors. Thus, in addition to the known benefits of salt reduction on reducing blood pressure, a reduction in salt intake in children may assist in reducing the amount of sugar-sweetened beverages consumed, which in turn may help to reduce energy intake and could be useful in obesity prevention efforts.

Longitudinal evaluation of milk type consumed and weight status in preschoolers

Scharf RJ[1], Demmer RT[2], DeBoer MD[1]

[1]Division of Developmental Pediatrics, Department of Pediatrics, University of Virginia School of Medicine, Charlottesville, VA, USA; [2]Department of Epidemiology, Mailman School of Public Health, Columbia University, New York, NY, USA

Arch Dis Child 2013; 98: 335–340

Background: The American Academy of Pediatrics recommends that children ≥2 years old consume low-fat milk. Data have been mixed regarding the associations between consumption of low-fat milk, weight status and weight gain over time in preschoolers.

Objective: It was hypothesized that low-fat milk would be associated with lower BMI z-score and less weight gain over time. Thus the aim of the study was to evaluate the relationship between milk fat consumption and BMI among a large cohort of preschool children.

Methods: In this longitudinal cohort study, a representative sample of US children, 10,700 children were examined at age 2 and 4 years. The BMI z-score and overweight/obese status as a function of milk type intake were assessed.

Results: The majority of children drank whole or 2% milk (87% at 2 years, 79.3% at 4 years). Drinkers of 1%/skim milk had higher BMI z-scores than 2%/whole-milk drinkers. In multivariable analyses, increasing fat content in the type of milk consumed was inversely associated with BMI z-score (p < 0.0001). Children 2 and 4 years old drinking 1%/skim milk compared to those drinking 2%/whole milk had an increased adjusted odds of being overweight (age 2, OR 1.64, p < 0.0001; age 4, OR 1.63, p < 0.0001) or obese (age 2, OR 1.57, p < 0.01; age 4, OR 1.64, p < 0.0001). In longitudinal analysis, children drinking 1%/skim milk at both 2 and 4 years were more likely to become over-weight/obese in this time period (adjusted OR 1.57, p < 0.05).

Conclusions: Consumption of low-fat milk did not prevent weight gain in preschoolers over time and was associated with an increased risk of overweight/obesity between 2 and 4 years of age.

Comments   In both children and adults, key contributors to the current obesity epidemic are the high-fat diets increasingly consumed worldwide. The AAP first started recommending low-fat milk for all children >2 years old in 2005 [9] after the onset of the current epidemic of obesity. Encouraging consumption of low-fat/skim milk instead of high-fat milk promotes a reduction of daily consumed fat and calories among children drinking milk. Using a large, nationally representative database, the researchers of this study found multiple associations between intake of 1%/skim milk and higher BMI z-scores in preschoolers, even across racial/ethnic and SES categories. These data may reflect the fact that parents of children with higher BMIs are more likely to adhere to recommendations of healthcare providers in selecting low-fat milk. Nevertheless, the prevalence of consumption of 1%/skim milk in preschool children remains low, as less than 20% of overweight or obese children consumed 1% or skim milk. Thus, healthcare practitioners following preschool children will have to focus on weight-control practices with a stronger evidence base than available for consumption of low-fat milk in order to reduce the risk of obesity.

Meal frequencies modify the effect of common genetic variants on body mass index in adolescents of the northern Finland birth cohort 1986

Jääskeläinen A[1], Schwab U[1,2], Kolehmainen M[1], Kaakinen M[3,4], Savolainen MJ[3,5,6], Froguel P[7-10], Cauchi S[8-10], Järvelin MR[3,4,11-13], Laitinen J[14]

[1]Department of Clinical Nutrition, Institute of Public Health and Clinical Nutrition, University of Eastern Finland, Kuopio, Finland; [2]Institute of Clinical Medicine, Internal Medicine, Kuopio University Hospital, Kuopio, Finland; [3]Biocenter Oulu, University of Oulu, Oulu, Finland; [4]Institute of Health Sciences, University of Oulu, Oulu, Finland; [5]Institute of Clinical Medicine, University of Oulu, Oulu, Finland; [6]Clinical Research Center, Department of Internal Medicine, Oulu University Hospital, Oulu, Finland; [7]Department of Genomics of Common Disease, School of Public Health, Imperial College London, London, UK; [8]CNRS UMR 8199, Lille Pasteur Institute, Lille, France; [9]Lille II University, Lille, France; [10]European Genomic Institute for Diabetes (EGID), Lille, France; [11]Department of Children and Young People and Families, National Institute for Health and Welfare, Oulu, Finland; [12]Department of Epidemiology and Biostatistics, MRC-HPA Centre for Environment and Health, School of Public Health, Imperial College London, London, UK; [13]Unit of Primary Care, Oulu University Hospital, Oulu, Finland; [14]Finnish Institute of Occupational Health, Oulu, Finland

PLoS One 2013; 8: e73802

Background: Several obesity-related genetic loci have been identified through genome-wide association studies (GWAS) in adult populations, with common single nucleotide polymorphisms (SNPs) in the *FTO* and *MC4R* genes also associated with weight gain in children and adolescents. Interestingly, behavioral modification can influence genetic risk: dietary fat composition was found to modify the association between the *FTO* gene variant rs9939609 and obesity risk in pediatric population, and in highly physically active adolescents the risk of higher BMI was significantly attenuated even among those carrying two risk alleles in the *FTO* gene.

Aims: The aim of the present study was to investigate the impact of two meal frequencies, 5 meals a day and <4 meals a day, on the association between obesity-related genotypes and BMI among adolescents.

Methods: From the prospective Finish neonatal cohort, 80% (n = 7,344) of the adolescents responded to a postal questionnaire concerning their health behavior and wellbeing and 74% (n = 6,798) participated in a clinical examination at the 16-year follow-up. Eight SNPs were genotyped at or near the *FTO* (fat mass- and obesity-associated), *MC4R* (melanocortin-4 receptor), *BDNF* (brain-derived neurotrophic factor), *GNPDA2* (glucosamine-6-phosphate deaminase-2), *MAF* (v-maf musculoaponeurotic fibrosarcoma oncogene homolog), *TMEM18* (transmembrane protein-18), *KCTD15* (potassium channel tetramerization domain containing-15), and *NEGR1* (neuronal growth regulator-1) genes, respectively.

Results: Carriers of two risk alleles in FTO rs1421085 had an increased BMI (21.7 [95% CI 21.5, 22.0] kg/m^2) compared with individuals with 0 or 1 risk allele (20.9 [95% CI 20.8, 21.1] kg/m^2 and 21.2 [95% CI 21.0, 21.3] kg/m^2, respectively). Similarly, carrying both of the risk-conferring alleles of rs17782313 at the MC4R locus was associated with a greater BMI (22.2 [95% CI 21.6, 22.9] kg/m^2) compared with the other two genotypes (TT 21.1 [95% CI 21.0, 21.2] kg/m^2 and CT 21.3 [95% CI 21.1, 21.5] kg/m^2). Regular meals were associated with lower BMI (20.7 [95% CI 20.6, 20.8] kg/m^2) as compared to skipping meals (21.6 [95% CI 21.5, 21.7] kg/m^2). The difference in BMI between the individuals with a high GRS (>8 BMI-increasing alleles) and those with a low GRS (<8 BMI increasing alleles) was 0.90 (95% CI 0.63, 1.17) kg/m^2 with irregular meals, whereas with the regular meals, this difference was only 0.32 (95% CI 0.06, 0.57) kg/m^2 (p interaction = 0.003). Moreover, gender-stratified analysis demonstrated significant interaction between the FTO rs1421085 and meal frequencies on BMI in boys (p interaction = 0.015) but not in girls (p interaction = 0.617). The difference in BMI between the carriers of the two MC4R rs17782313 risk alleles and non-carriers was elevated to 1.92 kg/m^2 with irregular meals, and reduced to 0.34 kg/m^2 (p interaction = 0.016) with irregular meals.

Conclusions: Each additional BMI-increasing allele was associated with an increase in BMI of 0.21 kg/m^2 which corresponds to a 0.61-kg increase in body weight for a person of 170 cm height. This was attenuated to 0.15 kg/m^2 (0.43 kg) with regular eating and increased to 0.27 kg/m^2 (0.78 kg) with irregular eating.

Comments This interesting study indicates that a regular five-meal-a-day habit tempers the effects of genetic susceptibility to increased BMI. Promoting a regular eating habit consisting of five meals including breakfast seems to be a powerful obesity prevention approach conveying additional important health benefits. We all are expecting confirmatory results, ideally from national large-scale randomized controlled intervention trials.

Eating frequency and overweight and obesity in children and adolescents: a meta-analysis

Kaisari P, Yannakoulia M, Panagiotakos DB

Department of Nutrition and Dietetics, Harokopio University, Athens, Greece

Pediatrics 2013; 131: 958–967

Background: The existing dietary etiological models cannot fully explain the development and maintenance of childhood obesity. Dietary patterns and eating behaviors may contribute to this epidemic more than consumption of specific nutrients and foods.

Objectives: The research question addressed here was to evaluate to what extent eating frequency is associated with body weight status (overweight/obesity), in children and adolescents. Total eating frequency was evaluated since there is no scientific consensus on the most appropriate definition to categorize the different eating occasions (i.e. meals vs. snacks).

Methods: Original research, observational studies published until October 2011, examining the association between eating frequency and overweight/obesity status in children and adolescents, were selected through a literature search in the PubMed database for this meta-analysis. Specific key words were used for this search: 'eating frequency', 'meal frequency', 'meals' and 'eating episodes,' in combination with the term 'overweight' or 'obesity' in children and adolescents. Pooled effect sizes were calculated using a random effects model.

Results: The presented meta-analysis of 21 substudies, with an overall incorporated population of 18,849 participants (aged 2–19 years), revealed an inverse association between eating frequency (i.e. the total number of meals/eating episodes consumed on a daily basis) and overweight/obesity status in children and adolescents. Specifically, children and adolescents who had a higher number of eating episodes per day had 22% lower probabilities of being overweight or obese compared with those who had fewer episodes. Interestingly, the inverse association was evident only in boys, suggesting that there are gender-related differences in dietary patterns and behaviors with their effect on overweight/obesity.

Conclusions: An inverse association was found between eating frequency and overweight/obesity status in children and adolescents. Gender-related differences emerged when this association was assessed separately in boys and girls, as the effect of eating frequency was only evident in boys.

Comments   Several pathways have been proposed to explain the association between higher eating frequency and lower body weight in children. In adults, it was found that increased eating frequency attenuates a series of postprandial metabolic and endocrine responses to dietary intake. The presented results are in accordance with a previous cross-sectional study in Greek adolescents, showing that the daily frequency of eating episodes was associated with obesity indices in boys, but not in girls [10]. However, it has to be emphasized that the subanalysis in girls was underpowered, and there was heterogeneity of the effect sizes of the selected studies leading to the inconsistencies between studies. Other limitations of this meta-analysis include: a significant heterogeneity in the pooled analysis, which caveats the generalization of the results, the methodological differences between studies, and the difference in the definition used for overweight/obesity in children and adolescents and the way that eating frequency was assessed, and finally confounding factors that were included in the analysis that varied between studies. Therefore, additional clinical trials are warranted to clarify potential mechanisms that may be responsible for a gender-dependent effect, to evaluate the clinical practice applicability, and support a public health recommendation.

Future studies should also evaluate the size and types of meals and snacks in terms of volume, energy content, macronutrient composition, or glycemic index and take this evaluation into account when investigating the associations between eating/meal patterns and obesity.

Identification of a dietary pattern prospectively associated with increased adiposity during childhood and adolescence

Ambrosini GL[1], Emmett PM[2], Northstone K[2], Howe LD[2], Tilling K[2], Jebb SA[1]

[1]Medical Research Council (MRC) Human Nutrition Research, Cambridge, UK; [2]School of Social and Community Medicine, University of Bristol, Bristol, UK

Int J Obes 2012; 36: 1299–1305

Background: Dietary intake is an important determinant of energy balance, but it is difficult to accurately measure energy intake (EI) in large population studies. Estimated EI is prone to dietary underreporting regardless of the dietary assessment method. The resulting imprecision in EI measurement makes it difficult to identify associations between EI and weight gain. Dietary pattern (DP) analyses have been increasingly used to consider total food intake and the potentially synergistic effects of foods and nutrients. Studies in adults suggest that dietary energy density, fat and fiber are critical dietary factors.

Objective: It was hypothesized that the same energy-dense, high-fat, low-fiber DP would be observed at 7, 10 and 13 years of age, and that this pattern would be prospectively associated with greater body fatness at 11, 13 and 15 years of age. As innate appetite control is stronger at younger ages, a second hypothesis was that the relationship between this DP and body fatness would strengthen with age. The longitudinal relationships between a DP characterized by dietary energy density, % total energy from fat and fiber density and fat mass (FM) was examined in children.

Methods: Children aged 7–15 years of age from the UK Avon Longitudinal Study of Parents and Children (n = 6,772) participated in the study. Their dietary intake was assessed using a 3-day food diary at 7, 10 and 13 years of age. An energy-dense, high-fat, low-fiber DP was identified using reduced rank regression and subjects scored for the DP at each age. Fat mass (FM) was measured at 11, 13 and 15 years and fat mass index (FMI) calculated as FM/height (χ).

Results: Girls had a higher prevalence of overweight or obesity based on BMI, at all ages. An increasing score for the energy-dense, high-fat, low-fiber DP at 7 years of age was associated with greater intakes of dietary energy density, % energy from fat and saturated fat, and lower fiber density, % energy from protein and carbohydrate, vitamin C and folate. Associations were similar at 10 and 13 years of age. DP z-scores at all ages were positively associated with later FMI. For each 1 SD unit increase in DP z-score, the odds of being in the highest quintile for FMI (as a marker of excess adiposity) increased by 13% (95% CI 1–27).

Conclusions: This analysis indicates that a DP that is high in energy density, high in fat and low in fiber is prospectively associated with greater adiposity in childhood and adolescence.

Comments   This study has several major strengths. Data were collected approximately every 2 years, enabling a longitudinal analysis spanning 7–15 years of age. The use of 3-day food diaries provides detailed characterization of dietary intake and avoids reliance on dietary recall. The observed associations between the DP and adiposity in this study were independent of physical activity measured objectively with accelerometers, whereas most other studies have relied on physical activity questionnaires. Therefore, this study provides important information for possible interventions and policy in the area of obesity prevention in young people.

Beneficial effects of a higher-protein breakfast on the appetitive, hormonal, and neural signals controlling energy intake regulation in overweight/obese, 'breakfast-skipping,' late-adolescent girls

Leidy HJ, Ortinau LC, Douglas SM, Hoertel HA

Department of Nutrition and Exercise Physiology, School of Medicine, University of Missouri, Columbia, MO, USA

Am J Clin Nutr 2013; 97: 677–688

Background: Recent evidence has isolated several key factors that play a critical role in the etiology of obesity, including the unhealthy dietary habit of breakfast skipping. In addition, breakfast skippers have poor diet quality and make poor food choices (e.g. snacking on nutrient-poor, high-fat, and/or high-sugar foods and beverages) compared with breakfast consumers. A diet rich in high-quality protein is considered a successful strategy to promote weight loss and/or prevent weight gain or regain in adults by improvement in appetite control and satiety. A protein-rich breakfast has been shown to reduce pre-lunch neural activation in brain regions that control food motivation/reward compared with skipping breakfast or consuming a normal-protein breakfast.

Objective: To examine in overweight/obese teenage girls who skip breakfast whether a high-protein (HP) breakfast leads to daily improvements in appetite control, satiety, food motivation/reward, and evening snacking compared with normal protein (NP) breakfast meals.

Methods: 20 overweight or obese teenage girls (mean age 19 ± 1 years, BMI 28.6 ± 0.7) who skip breakfast participated in this randomized crossover study. The participants randomly completed the following breakfast patterns at home for 6 days: (1) breakfast skipping, (2) consumption of 350-kcal NP breakfast meals cereal-based (13 g protein), or (3) consumption of 350-kcal HP breakfast meals egg- and beef-rich (35 g protein). On the 7th day of each pattern, a standardized NP lunch was provided 4 h after breakfast, and a 10-hour testing was completed that included appetite and satiety questionnaires, blood sampling, pre-dinner food cue-stimulated functional MRI brain scans, ad libitum dinner, and evening snacking.

Results: The consumption of breakfast reduced daily hunger compared with breakfast skipping with no differences between meals. Breakfast, especially that containing HP, increased daily fullness, and reduced evening snacking of high-fat foods compared with breakfast skipping. HP breakfast also reduced daily ghrelin and increased daily peptide YY concentrations compared with breakfast skipping. Both meals reduced pre-dinner amygdala, hippocampal, and midfrontal corticolimbic activation compared with breakfast skipping.

Conclusions: The consumption of 350-kcal breakfast meals led to daily reductions in perceived hunger, desire to eat, and prospective food consumption; daily increases in perceived fullness, and reduced dinner-time neural activation in selected cortico-limbic brain regions that control food motivation/reward in overweight/obese breakfast-skipping teens. Additional benefits were observed with the consumption of the HP breakfast compared with the NP cereal-based version with greater increases in daily perceived fullness and greater reductions in cortico-limbic activation compared with the NP breakfast, daily reductions in the hunger-stimulating hormone ghrelin, increases in the satiety hormone PYY, and reductions in evening snacking, particularly of high-fat foods, compared with skipping breakfast. Thus, the addition of breakfast, particularly one rich in protein, might be an important dietary strategy to improve satiety, reduce food motivation/reward, and improve diet quality in overweight/obese teen girls.

Comments   Young people consume nearly half of their daily calories between 16:00 and 24:00 h; the snack foods often craved and consumed consist of highly palatable, but calorically dense foods with little nutritional value. These habits contribute substantially to the shift away from eating according to physiologic need toward reward-driven eating which leads to positive energy balance and obesity. Skipping breakfast exacerbates the desire to snack. Adolescents who skip breakfast typically snack on more desserts, high-fat salty foods, and sodas compared with breakfast consumers. The consumption of dietary protein appears to modulate key gastrointestinal hormones, which provide signals to the central, homeostatic, neuronal pathways to alter appetite, satiety, and regulate energy intake. The current study design allowed exploring sustained effects over the course of an 8-hour day. Only the HP breakfast led to sustained alterations in perceived desire to eat, prospective food consumption, fullness, and reduced plasma ghrelin into the afternoon periods, with elevated plasma PYY throughout the morning and afternoon periods. These data support the role of increased dietary protein at the morning meal to provide immediate and/or sustained improvements in the appetitive and hormonal signals that control food intake regulation. The HP breakfast also led to reduced amygdala, hippocampus, and midfrontal activation compared with skipping breakfast, and to reduced hippocampus and parahippocampal activation compared with the NP breakfast. These findings suggest that an HP breakfast affects homeostatic and non-homeostatic reward signals that control food intake regulation in teen girls.

Optimal macronutrient content of the diet for adolescents with pre-diabetes: RESIST a randomized control trial

Garnett SP[1,5], Gow M[1,5], Ho M[5], Baur LA[5], Noakes M[6], Woodhead HJ[7,8], Broderick CR[2], Burrell S[3], Chisholm K[3], Halim J[1], De S, Steinbeck K[9], Srinivasan S[1], Ambler GR[1,5], Kohn MR[4], Cowell CT[1,5]

[1]Institute of Endocrinology and Diabetes, [2]The Children's Hospital Institute of Sports Medicine, [3]Nutrition and Dietetics, Weight Management Services, [4]The Centre for Research into Adolescent's Health, [5]The Children's Hospital at Westmead, The Children's Hospital at Westmead Clinical School, [6]University of Sydney, Westmead, NSW, Australia; Commonwealth Scientific and Industrial Research Organisation Food and Nutritional Sciences; [7]Adelaide Business Centre, Adelaide, SA, Australia; [8]Department of Paediatrics, Campbelltown Hospital, Campbelltown, NSW, Australia; [9]Department of Diabetes and Endocrinology, Sydney Children's Hospital Network, Randwick, NSW, Australia and Academic Department of Adolescent Medicine, Sydney Medical School, University of Sydney, NSW, Australia

J Clin Endocrinol Metab 2013; 98: 2116–2125

Background: Insulin resistance and glucose intolerance are considered as continuous parameters that increase the likelihood of developing type 2 diabetes. Current methods of dietary intervention in children and adolescents for weight management include the traffic light diet, a hypocaloric diet or general healthy eating advice. An alternative approach is a moderate-carbohydrate, increased-protein diet.

Objective: The aim of this trial was to determine the effectiveness of two different structured lifestyle interventions differing in diet composition on insulin sensitivity, anthropometry, and cardiometabolic profile in adolescents with pre-diabetes and/or clinical features of insulin resistance treated with metformin.

Methods: This was a randomized controlled trial of overweight or obese children and adolescents aged 10 to 17 years with either pre-diabetes and/or clinical features of insulin resistance. Participants were prescribed metformin and randomized to a structured isocaloric diet, which was either high carbohydrate or moderate carbohydrate with increased protein. The program commenced with a 3-month dietary intervention, with the addition of physical activity intervention in the next 3 months.

Results: 111 subjects (66 girls) were recruited and 98 subjects (58 girls) completed the 6-month intervention. At baseline significantly more participants had pre-diabetes in the increased-protein diet group compared with those in the high-carbohydrate diet group (11 and 3, p < 0.024, respectively). No other significant differences were observed in other baseline parameters between the intervention groups. After 3 months of dietary intervention and treatment with metformin, there were significant decreases in the BMI 95th percentile and waist-to-height ratio (both p < 0.001) and there was an estimated mean increase in insulin sensitivity index (ISI) of 0.3 (95% CI 0.2–0.4). At 6 months, BMI 95th percentile and waist-to-height ratio remained significantly different from baseline. The insulin-to-glucose ratio decreased over the first 3 months and remained statistically different from the baseline measures at 6 months, with an estimated mean decrease of 7.2 (95% CI 2.3–12.0). No significant differences were observed between the diet groups at any time point, and there was no significant change over time in the lipid profile in either diet group. Systolic BP (SBP) z-scores and diastolic BP (DBP) z-scores decreased over 3 months and remained significantly lower at 6 months compared with baseline, without a difference between diet groups at any time point.

Conclusions: In adolescents at high risk of developing type 2 diabetes, a 6-month lifestyle intervention with metformin can achieve modest weight loss and increased insulin sensitivity. Many adolescents had difficulty adhering to their prescribed diets and the diets had no differential effect on change in ISI or the BMI 95th percentile relative to one another. Further strategies are required to better address pre-diabetes and the clinical features of insulin resistance in adolescents.

Comments The lack of observed differences in outcomes between dietary groups may be due to poor or variable dietary adherence or limitations of monitoring and reporting in both groups. Many of the adolescents had difficulty adhering to their prescribed diet, and few were able to reach the target protein or carbohydrate intake. The lack of improvement in insulin sensitively and weight loss observed in this study during the exercise program is consistent with a recent systematic review that concluded that the addition of exercise to a dietary intervention does not result in greater weight loss in overweight and obese adolescents [11]. However, it is possible that the exercise program prevented weight gain. The limitations of the study include: lack of data about dietary intake measurements at baseline, with inability to determine whether the energy intake was altered by either intervention; the measures of dietary compliance that were based on a standardized 24-hour recall and non-blinding of participants and dietitians who implemented the dietary intervention. Further strategies are required to better address pre-diabetes and the clinical features of insulin resistance in adolescents.

Childhood nutrition in predicting metabolic syndrome in adults: the cardiovascular risk in Young Finns Study

Jääskeläinen P[1], Magnussen CG[1,2], Pahkala K[1], Mikkilä V[3], Kähönen M[4], Sabin MA[5], Fogelholm M[3], Hutri-Kähönen N[6], Taittonen L[7,8], Telama R[9], Laitinen T[10], Jokinen E[11], Lehtimäki T[12], Viikari JSA[13], Raitakari OT[1,14] Juonala M[1,13]

[1]Research Centre of Applied and Preventive Cardiovascular Medicine, University of Turku, Turku, Finland; [2]Menzies Research Institute Tasmania, University of Tasmania, Hobart, TAS, Australia; [3]Department of Food and Environmental Sciences, University of Helsinki, Helsinki, Finland; [4]Department of Clinical Physiology, Tampere University Hospital and University of Tampere, School of Medicine, Tampere, Finland; [5]Murdoch Children's Research Institute, Melbourne, VIC, Australia; [6]Department of Pediatrics, Tampere University Hospital and University of Tampere, School of Medicine, Tampere, Finland; [7]Department of Pediatrics, Vaasa Central Hospital, Vaasa, Finland; [8]Department of Pediatrics, University of Oulu, Oulu, Finland; [9]Department of Sport Sciences, University of Jyväskylä, Jyväskylä, Finland; [10]Department of Clinical Physiology, Kuopio University Hospital and University of Eastern Finland, Kuopio, Finland; [11]Hospital for Children and Adolescents, University of Helsinki, Helsinki, Finland; [12]Department of Clinical Chemistry, Tampere University Hospital and University of Tampere, School of Medicine, Tampere, Finland; [13]Department of Medicine, University of Turku and Turku University Hospital, Turku, Finland; [14]Department of Clinical Physiology, University of Turku and Turku University Hospital, Turku, Finland

Diabetes Care 2012; 35: 1937–1943

Background: The metabolic syndrome (MetS) is a major medical and public health problem that has increased in prevalence during the past decades. It represents a clustering of interrelated cardiometabolic risk factors, including obesity, hypertension, dyslipidemia, hyperglycemia, and hyperinsulinemia. In adults, the vegetarian dietary pattern has been shown to have a beneficial effect on metabolic risk factors and to lower the risk of MetS.

Objective: The aim of the study was to examine the associations between childhood lifestyle factors (i.e. the frequency of certain food consumption and physical activity) and MetS in adulthood.

Methods: The study cohort included 2,128 individuals from the Cardiovascular Risk in Young Finns Study participating in the baseline study in 1980 (3–18 years of age) and the 27-year follow-up in 2007. The average of lifestyle factor measurements taken in 1980, 1983, and 1986 in the analyses were used. Childhood dietary factors and physical activity were assessed by self-reported questionnaires.

Results: Participants with MetS had lower HDL cholesterol, were more males than females, and had higher age, triglycerides, systolic blood pressure, CRP, insulin, and BMI in childhood than those without MetS. The difference was significant for all risk variables, with the exception of LDL cholesterol. Those who had adult MetS reported having less consumption of fruit and vegetables than those who did not have adult MetS. There were no significant differences in physical activity index, fish consumption, meat consumption, and butter use between these two groups. Childhood vegetable consumption frequency was inversely associated with adult MetS (OR 0.86, p = 0.02) in a multivariable analysis adjusted with age, gender, childhood metabolic risk factors (lipids, systolic blood pressure, insulin, BMI, and C-reactive protein), family history of type 2 diabetes and hypertension, and socioeconomic status. Decreased frequency of childhood vegetable consumption predicted high blood pressure (OR 0.88, p = 0.01) and a high triglyceride value (OR 0.88, p = 0.03) after adjustment for the above-mentioned risk factors.

Conclusions: Childhood vegetable consumption frequency had a significant inverse association with adult MetS after adjustment for several lifestyle and traditional risk factors. Every effort to support a healthy lifestyle in childhood is needed to prevent the increase in the prevalence of MetS.

Comments Previous studies have shown that childhood obesity, high triglycerides, high insulin, high CRP, and family history of type 2 diabetes and hypertension were determinants of adult MetS during the 21-year follow-up. Rizzo et al. [12] reported that a vegetarian dietary pattern had a favorable effect on metabolic risk factors and lowered the risk of MetS. Higher intakes of vegetables and fruit and dietary patterns rich in these foods, as in the Mediterranean diet, have also been associated with a lower risk of MetS in several studies [13]. Food choices and physical activity are established early in childhood and these behaviors may track into adulthood. Multiple risk factors for cardiovascular diseases have also been shown to cluster already in young adults. Therefore, it appears important to focus on dietary education in childhood if the prevention of the development of these adverse risk factors is to be maximized. It seems that a child should eat vegetables every day or almost every day at all ages to get the protective effect of vegetables against the MetS in adulthood. The strength of this study was the large, randomly selected study population of young men and women who were prospectively followed up for 27 years since childhood. Surprisingly, there was a lack of association between adult MetS and the traditional lifestyle factors: total caloric intake, diet composition, and physical activity in childhood.

Correcting vitamin D insufficiency improves insulin sensitivity in obese adolescents: a randomized controlled trial

Belenchia AM[1], Tosh AK[2], Hillman LS[2], Peterson CA[1]

[1]Department of Nutrition and Exercise Physiology and [2]Department of Child Health, University of Missouri School of Medicine, University of Missouri, Columbia, MO, USA

Am J Clin Nutr 2013; 97: 774–781

Background: Obese adolescents may have vitamin D deficiency due to poor-quality nutrition and vitamin D sequestration in excessive adipose tissue. Low vitamin D concentrations are associated with a higher prevalence of the metabolic syndrome or/and type 2 diabetes.

Aims: The efficacy and safety of 4,000 IU vitamin D_3 daily in obese adolescents was investigated in a randomized controlled trial.

Methods: The efficacy and safety of 4,000 IU vitamin D_3 daily in obese adolescents was investigated in a randomized controlled trial. Circulating concentrations of 25-hydroxyvitamin D [25(OH)D] were determined and association with markers of insulin sensitivity, resistance and inflammation were investigated. 35 obese adolescents [mean ± SD age 14.1 ± 2.8 years; BMI 39.8 ± 6.1 kg/m^2; 25(OH)D 19.4 ± 7.3 ng/ml] were recruited and randomly assigned to receive either vitamin D_3 (4,000 IU/days) or placebo as part of their standard care. Anthropometric measurements, inflammatory markers (IL-6, TNF-α, C-reactive protein), adipokines (leptin, adiponectin), fasting glucose, fasting insulin, and HOMA-IR values were measured at baseline, and after 3 and 6 months of follow-up.

Results: No significant differences between groups in BMI, serum inflammatory markers, or plasma glucose concentrations were appreciated at 6 months. Vitamin D_3 supplementation increased serum 25(OH)D concentrations (to 38.9 ng/ml compared to 22.2 ng/ml for placebo; $p < 0.001$), fasting insulin (−6.5 compared with +1.2 μU/ml for placebo; $p = 0.026$), HOMA-IR (−1.363 compared with +0.27 for placebo; $p = 0.033$), QUICKI (−0.016 compared with −0.004 for placebo; $p = 0.016$) and leptin-to-adiponectin ratio (−1.41 compared with +0.10 for placebo; $p = 0.045$). There was a significant negative linear correlation between serum 25(OH)D concentrations and leptin-to-adiponectin ratio ($p < 0.01$).

Conclusions: Supplementing vitamin D to obese adolescents may be an effective strategy for reducing insulin resistance in addition to the standard treatment for obesity.

Comments   The study was conducted in a very limited population and as such adds to the controversy of the efficacy of vitamin D supplementation in obesity and pre-diabetes. Fifteen vitamin D trials were included in a recent systematic review [14]: no significant improvement was seen in fasting glucose, HbA_{1c} or insulin resistance in those supplemented with vitamin D compared to placebo when all studies were combined. Meta-analysis for patients with impaired glucose tolerance or diabetes indicated a small effect on fasting glucose (–0.32 mmol/l, 95% CI –0.57 to –0.07) and insulin resistance (standard mean difference –0.25, 95% CI –0.48 to –0.03). No effect was seen HbA_{1c} in patients with diabetes and no differences were seen for any outcome in patients with normal fasting glucose. It is therefore difficult to propose a universal supplementation of vitamin D to all people with obesity, however a larger well-designed and controlled trial in pre-diabetes and diabetes is warranted.

Probiotics to adolescents with obesity: effects on inflammation and metabolic syndrome

Gøbel RJ[1], Larsen N[2], Jakobsen M[2], Mølgaard C[1], Michaelsen KF[1]

[1]Department of Human Nutrition and [2]Department of Food Science, Faculty of Sciences, University of Copenhagen, Frederiksberg, Denmark

J Pediatr Gastroenterol Nutr 2012; 55: 673–678

Background: Evidence from animal studies indicates that the composition of the gut microbiota is involved in extraintestinal disorders such as obesity. The connection between gut microbiota, energy homeostasis, and inflammation, and its role in the pathogenesis of obesity-related disorders are increasingly recognized. Despite this, studies investigating the effect of probiotics on obesity-related inflammation are few and mainly based on animal models.

Objective: To investigate the effect of the probiotic strain, *Lactobacillus salivarius* Ls-33, on biomarkers related to inflammation and the metabolic syndrome in adolescents with obesity.

Methods: This was a double-blind, randomized, placebo-controlled intervention study including 50 obese 12- to 15-year-old adolescents. Participants were randomized to receive a daily dose of either *L. salivarius* Ls-33 ATCC SD5208 (10^{10} CFU) or placebo daily for 12 weeks.

Results: 14% of the adolescents fulfilled the criteria for metabolic syndrome. There were no differences between the groups at baseline in BMI *z*-score, waist/hip ratio, body fat percentage, blood pressure or metabolic and inflammatory biomarkers. Compliance based on calculation of remaining capsules and self-reported diaries was ~91.3%. The BMI z-score did not change significantly in either of the groups from baseline to after intervention. Concentrations of fasting insulin, HOMA-IR, and C-peptide decreased significantly and FFA increased significantly from baseline to after intervention in the placebo group, without a significant difference compared with the Ls-33 intervention group. There were no differences in change for any of the inflammatory markers, adjusted for baseline values, from baseline to after intervention between the groups. *L. salivarius* was detected in 89% of the subjects of the probiotic group after intake of Ls-33 at the mean level of 5.55 ($\pm$0.95) $\log_{10}$ cells per gram stool.

Conclusions: No effects of the intervention with the probiotic strain Ls-33 on either the inflammatory markers or the markers of metabolic syndrome were found.

Comments   It is estimated that the gut microbiota contains, at least, 100-fold more genes than the mammalian genome. These bacteria can live in a symbiotic way but, in certain cases, promote disease. In the last decade, a great body of evidence and knowledge about the gut microbiota and its interaction with the host, immunity, energy metabolism and insulin sensitivity has provided new insights regarding the influence of this forgotten 'organ' on the most prevalent metabolic disease, obesity. Gut bacteria influence the chronic low-grade inflammation that culminates in insulin resistance and the increase in fat deposition and body weight gain, characteristic of obese individuals. The issue of the 'healthy' bacterial group profile is a very important point in gut microbiota research and needs to be further explored. Thus, no proposed treatment attempting to induce the proliferation of certain bacterial phyla has been suggested until now. Probiotics are defined as live microorganisms that confer unspecified health benefits to the host. Evidence from metagenomic profiles indicates that the obese phenotype shows an increased prevalence of *Firmicutes* [15] in the gut microbiota profile, inferring a negative correlation with metabolism and insulin sensitivity. The most commonly used probiotics are *Lactobacillus*, which belong to *Firmicutes* and *Bifidobacterium*. Although the mechanism by which *Lactobacillus* control excessive adiposity has not been described, changes in fat storage genes expression have been proposed to mediate this probiotic effect. The recent study failed to demonstrate a beneficial effect of the probiotic intervention on inflammatory markers or parameters related to the metabolic syndrome, which may be explained by the reality that results from in vitro and animal studies could not be translated to humans for this strain. The negative results of the probiotic impact might also be affected by the amount of daily administrated probiotic that was not enough to get a significant impact, or the relatively short period of administration and follow-up. However, we also cannot exclude that other strains of bacteria will have beneficial effects in populations with high levels of risk factors for obesity-related comorbidities. Therefore, more studies, especially randomized controlled trials, within this research area are needed.

Role of carbohydrate modification in weight management among obese children: a randomized clinical trial

Kirk S[1], Brehm B[2], Saelens BE[3], Woo JG[1,4], Kissel E[5], D'Alessio D[6], Bolling C[7], Daniels SR[8]

[1]Center for Better Health and Nutrition, The Heart Institute, Cincinnati Children's Hospital Medical Center, Cincinnati, OH, USA; [2]College of Nursing, University of Cincinnati, Cincinnati, OH, USA; [3]Center for Child Health, Behavior and Development, Seattle Children's Research Institute, Seattle, WA, USA; [4]Division of Biostatistics and Epidemiology, Cincinnati Children's Hospital Medical Center, Cincinnati, OH, USA; [5]Good Samaritan Hospital, Department of Nutrition Services, Cincinnati, OH, USA; [6]Division of Endocrinology and Cincinnati Veterans Affairs Medical Center, University of Cincinnati, Cincinnati, OH, USA; [7]Division of General and Community Pediatrics, Cincinnati Children's Hospital Medical Center, Cincinnati, OH, USA; [8]University of Colorado School of Medicine, The Children's Hospital Colorado, Auroa, CO, USA

J Pediatrics 2012; 161: 320–327

Background: Effective weight management strategies for obese children became an important issue in pediatrics. Guidelines for pediatric weight management include increased physical activity, less sedentary time, and a nutritionally balanced diet, with an emphasis on fat and sugar restriction to limit caloric intake. However, the standard recommendations for achieving 'negative energy balance' are typically associated with only modest and transient improvements in weight status, often because of poor long-term adherence.

Objective: To compare the safety and efficacy of low-CHO (LC) and reduced glycemic load (RGL) diets and a standard portion-controlled (PC) dietary intervention for the management of obesity in young children aged 7–12 years.

Methods: Obese children (n = 102) were randomly assigned to a 3-month intervention of a LC, RGL, or standard PC diet, along with weekly dietary counseling and biweekly group exercise. Subjects in the LC diet group were instructed to limit CHO intake and to measure ketones daily. The subjects were instructed to follow a 2-week induction phase with ≤20 g CHO/day and unrestricted intake of high-protein foods and added fats. After induction, CHO intake was increased by 5–10 g/week up to a maximum of 60 g/day, with no limit on intake of high-protein foods and fats. Subjects in the RGL diet group were instructed to limit their intake of high-glycemic index (GI) foods. A 'stoplight approach' was modified to classify foods according to GI values ('red' foods, high GI: ≥70; 'yellow' foods, medium GI: 56–69; 'green' foods, low GI: ≤55). Green foods were not restricted. Yellow foods were to be consumed less frequently. Red foods were restricted to ≤7 servings/week and ≤2 servings/day. Subjects in the PC diet group were instructed to consume age-appropriate, PC amounts of grains, vegetables, fruits, lean proteins, and skim/low-fat dairy products. Calories were distributed as 55–60% CHO, 10–15% protein, and 30% fat. Anthropometry, dietary adherence, and clinical measures were evaluated at baseline and 3, 6, and 12 months.

Results: 85 children (83%) completed the 12-month assessment. Dietary adherence was consistently high in the RGL group (>75%), and adherence was significantly lower in the LC group than in the other two groups at all visits. At 3 months, body mass index z-score was lower in all diet groups (LC –0.27 ± 0.04; RGL –0.20 ± 0.04; PC –0.21 ± 0.04; $p < 0.0001$) and was maintained at 6 months, with similar results for waist circumference and percent of body fat. At 12 months, participants in all diet groups had lower BMI z-scores than at baseline (LC –0.21 ± 0.04; RGL –0.28 ± 0.04; PC –0.31 ± 0.04; $p < 0.0001$), and lower percent of body fat, but the reductions in waist circumference was not maintained. Despite similar overall energy intake, subjects in the different diet groups consumed diets with differing macronutrient compositions.

Conclusions: The 3 diets, which differed in macronutrient content and GL, resulted in similar and significant improvements in BMI z-score and related health measures in children. Although strict adherence to the LC diet was more difficult to achieve in children, all diets were effective in decreasing adiposity and improving clinical outcomes. These findings suggest that practitioners may offer any of these dietary approaches for achieving a healthier weight in obese children.

Comments   The results of the recent study do not support the hypothesis that CHO-modified diets would be more effective in improving weight status than a standard PC diet in obese children. Subjects in all 3 diet groups showed significant improvements in adiposity measures during the initial 3-month intervention with relatively intensive intervention and contact with study dietitians. At 12 months, improvements in BMI z-score and percent of body fat were maintained in all 3 diet groups, however none of the groups sustained improvements in waist circumference. Subjects in all 3 diet groups successfully maintained a reduced caloric intake and altered dietary composition even in the final 9 months without intervention contact. These findings raise the possibility that intensive guidance with the initial clinical application of weight management diets can lead to long-term success in children. Recently it has been suggested that strategies to individualize diet interventions to match patients' metabolic profiles could have increased efficacy [16]. This trial provides limited support for this hypothesis, with detection of differential effects on specific metabolic profiles (e.g. lipids vs. insulin resistance) by dietary intervention. The sustained high adherence to the RGL diet, coupled with anthropometric and clinical improvements, may make this diet the most promising intervention for the long-term weight management of children. Alternatively, prescribing one of the 3 diets based on the patient's preferences for the initial intervention and then transitioning to the RGL diet for longer-term maintenance may also be an effective strategy.

Summary: People usually describe food as either good or bad or something in between. The overview of the above recent publications provides evidence that food can be beneficial or dangerous to young people, particularly to those with certain genetic predispositions, and can in specific time-windows even determine several long-term risks. There is considerable confusion both in the professional and lay communities as the facts on nutrition are blurred with a conundrum of poorly controlled, poorly executed, observational or biased studies. Therefore, the aim of this overview was to shed some clear light on this extremely important field by discussing data from recent trials that addressed pertinent questions on nutrition of the young. An important message from the recent research in nutrition related to obesity and diabetes is that behavioral modification can defy our thrifty genes. We should find more successful ways to efficiently convey this scientific discovery to the minds of people.

References

1 Ogden CL, Carroll MD, Kit BK, Flegal KM: Prevalence of obesity and trends in body mass index among US children and adolescents, 1999–2010. JAMA 2012;307:483–490.

2 Whitaker RC, Wright JA, Pepe MS, Seidel KD, Dietz WH: Predicting obesity in young adulthood from childhood and parental obesity. N Engl J Med 1997; 337:869–873.

3 Chaput JP, Klingenberg L, Astrup A, Sjodin AM: Modern sedentary activities promote overconsumption of food in our current obesogenic environment. Obes Rev 2011;12:e12–e20.

4 Wardle J, Carnell S, Haworth CMA, Plomin R: Evidence for a strong genetic influence on childhood adiposity despite the force of the obesogenic environment. Am J Clin Nutr 2008;87:398–404.

5 Temple JL, Giacomelli AM, Kent KM, Roemmich JN, Epstein LH: Television watching increases motivated responding for food and energy intake in children. Am J Clin Nutr 2007;85:355–361.

6 Malik VS, Popkin BM, Bray GA, Despres JP, Hu FB: Sugar-sweetened beverages, obesity, type 2 diabetes mellitus, and cardiovascular disease risk. Circulation 2010;121:1356–1364.

7 Qi Q, Chu AY, Kang JH, Jensen MK, Curhan GC, Pasquale LR, Ridker PM, Hunter DJ, Willett WC, Rimm EB, Chasman DI, Hu FB, Qi L: Sugar-sweetened beverages and genetic risk of obesity. N Engl J Med 2012;367:1387–1396.

8 Malik VS, Popkin BM, Bray GA, Despres JP, Willett WC, Hu FB: Sugar-sweetened beverages and risk of metabolic syndrome and type 2 diabetes. A meta-analysis. Diabetes Care 2010;33:2477–2483.

9 Gidding SS, Dennison BA, Birch LL, et al: Dietary recommendations for children and adolescents: a guide for practitioners: consensus statement from the American Heart Association. Circulation 2005; 112:2061–2075.

10 Kosti RI, Panagiotakos DB, Mihas CC, et al: Dietary habits, physical activity and prevalence of overweight/obesity among adolescents in Greece: the Vyronas study. Med Sci Monit 2007;13:CR437–CR444.

11 Ho M, Garnett SP, Baur LA, et al: Effectiveness of lifestyle interventions in child obesity: a systematic review with meta-analysis. Pediatrics 2012;130: e1647–e1671.

12 Rizzo NS, Sabaté J, Jaceldo-Siegl K, Fraser GE: Vegetarian dietary patterns are associated with a lower risk of metabolic syndrome: the Adventist Health Study 2. Diabetes Care 2011;34:1225–1227.

13 Richard C, Couture P, Desroches S, Lamarche B: Effect of the Mediterranean diet with and without weight loss on markers of inflammation in men with metabolic syndrome. Obesity 2013;21:51–57.

14 George PS, Pearson ER, Witham MD: Effect of vitamin D supplementation on glycaemic control and insulin resistance: a systematic review and meta-analysis. Diabet Med 2012;29:e142–e150.

15 Caricilli AM, Picardi PK, de Abreu LL, et al: Gut microbiota is a key modulator of insulin resistance in TLR-2 knockout mice. PLOS Biol 2011;9:e1001212.

16 Ebbling CB, Leidig MM, Feldman HA, Lovesky MM, Ludwig DS: Effects of a low-glycemic load vs. low-fat diet in obese young adults. A randomized trial. JAMA 2007;297:2092–2102.

Battelino/Shalitin

Koletzko B, Shamir R, Turck D, Phillip M (eds): Nutrition and Growth: Yearbook 2014.
World Rev Nutr Diet. Basel, Karger, 2014, vol 109, pp 23–35 (DOI: 10.1159/000356106)

Neonatal and Infant Nutrition, Breastfeeding

Dominique Turck[1] and J.B. (Hans) van Goudoever[2,3]

[1]Division of Gastroenterology, Hepatology and Nutrition, Department of Pediatrics, Jeanne de Flandre
Children's Hospital and Lille University Faculty of Medicine; INSERM U995, Lille, France
[2]Department of Pediatrics, VU University Medical Center, Amsterdam, The Netherlands
[3]Department of Pediatrics, Emma Children's Hospital – Academic Medical Center, Amsterdam, The Netherlands

The period of infancy and young childhood is characterized by special needs in nutrition, which not only must maintain the body but also support a rapid rate of growth and the appropriate synthesis and deposition of body tissue. This growth leads to a doubling of the body weight at the age of 3–4 months and to a tripling at the age of 12 months. Moreover, the quantity and quality of nutrient supply during infancy and young childhood has been shown to be associated with long-term health effects, some of which being the consequences of 'programming' [1].

A special feature of young infancy is that one liquid food is the sole source of nutrition. Breast milk is the optimal food for all healthy infants and provides an adequate supply of nutrients to support a healthy growth and development (with the exception of vitamin K during the first weeks of life and of vitamin D), besides providing anti-infective protection and immunostimulatory components. Studies performed in affluent countries have shown important advantages of breastfeeding over formula feeding, such as lower incidence rates of gastrointestinal and respiratory infections and a lower risk of obesity. Breast milk is the model for the composition of infant formula taking into account that a breast milk substitute should not only imitate the composition of breast milk but also aim at achieving similar health effects [2].

This chapter of the *Yearbook on Nutrition and Growth* reviews the key articles that have appeared between 1 July 2012 and 30 June 2013 in the area of neonatal and infant nutrition, including breastfeeding. All studies were human observational or clinical trials. Comments are included following the summaries of papers. References used in the introduction and in the comments are listed at the end of the chapter.

Randomized trial of exclusive human milk versus preterm formula diet in extremely premature infants

Cristofalo EA[1], Schanler RJ[2], Blanco CL[3], Sullivan S[4], Trawöger R[5], Kiechl-Kohlendorfer U[5], Dudell G[6], Rechtman DJ[7], Lee ML[7], Lucas A[8], Abrams S[9]

[1]Department of Pediatrics, Johns Hopkins School of Medicine, Baltimore, MD, USA; [2]Division of Neonatal-Perinatal Medicine, Cohen Children's Medical Center of New York, New Hyde Park, NY, USA; [3]Department of Pediatrics, University of Texas Health Science Center, San Antonio, TX, USA; [4]Department of Pediatrics, University of Florida, Gainesville, FL, USA; [5]Department of Pediatrics, Innsbruck Medical University, Innsbruck, Austria; [6]Children's Hospital and Research Center, Oakland, CA, USA; [7]Prolacta Bioscience, Monrovia, CA, USA; [8]MRC Child Nutrition Research Center, Institute of Child Health, London, UK; [9]Department of Pediatrics, Baylor College of Medicine, Houston, TX, USA

J Pediatr 2013 (E-pub ahead of print)

Background: Own mother's milk is the preferred choice to feed premature infants enterally. Second choice is donor human milk, while preterm formula might be the alternative. While the use of human milk is associated with a reduction in nosocomial sepsis and necrotizing enterocolitis, large controlled studies of donor human milk on objective outcome criteria are lacking. The objective of this multicenter, randomized controlled trial was to compare the duration of parenteral nutrition, growth, and morbidity in extremely premature infants fed exclusive diets of either bovine milk-based preterm formula (BOV) or donor human milk and human milk-based human milk fortifier (HUM) of formula vs. human milk.

Methods: The study randomized 53 infants with a birth weight of 500–1,250 g whose mothers did not intend to provide milk, who received parenteral nutrition within 48 h after birth and enteral feedings before 21 days of age. Intervention consisted of an exclusive human milk diet of pasteurized donor human milk and human milk-based fortifier, compared to a bovine-based preterm formula. Study participation ended at the earliest of the following milestones: 91 days of age, discharge from the hospital (to home or to another hospital), or attainment of 50% oral feedings (i.e. 4 complete oral feedings per day). The major outcome was duration of parenteral nutrition. Secondary outcomes were growth, respiratory support, and necrotizing enterocolitis (NEC).

Results: This relatively small group of infants did not differ in birth weight (approx. 1,000 g) or gestational age (27–28 weeks). There was a significant difference in median parenteral nutrition days: 36 vs. 27 in formula-fed infants vs. donor human milk-fed infants, respectively (p = 0.04). The incidence of NEC in the formula-fed group was not significantly different but tended to be higher than in the donor human milk group (21% (5 cases) vs. 3% (1 case), p = 0.08). Surgical NEC was significantly higher in the formula-fed group (4 cases) than in the donor human milk group (0 cases), p = 0.04.

Conclusions: Feeding with exclusive diet of formula compared with human milk in extreme preterm infants resulted in longer duration of parenteral feeding and higher rate of surgical NEC. These findings support a greater need for enhanced lactation or use of exclusive human milk diet of preterm infants in the neonatal intensive care units.

Comments The use of a human milk-based diet in the neonatal intensive care unit has been advocated for some time. The present study shows that an important outcome, i.e. days on parenteral nutrition is significantly reduced when fed commercially available pasteurized donor human milk only. In an earlier study, an exclusively human milk-based diet, but including approximately 80% of own mother's milk, the same authors reported a significant reduction in NEC as well [3]. That study was severely criticized because of the high incidence of NEC in the control group. Again in this study the authors describe an incidence of 21%, much higher than in other studies reported in infants receiving formula only. The present study was powered to detect a reduction in parenteral nutrition days, which were significantly lower in the human milk group. The claim on NEC reduction is not appropriate as this was not the primary outcome. The results can only be seen as hypothesis-generating. Furthermore, the incidence of nosocomial infections is extremely high (55–79%), which is not discussed. However, there seemed to be such a trend. Many previous studies describe an association with reduced nosocomial infections when fed a human milk-based diet. That growth rates are low, which is associated with a less favorable neurocognitive outcome, might be overcome with a more appropriate fortification of the human milk-based fortifier. Nonetheless, the data are encouraging and warrant a large independent trial powered to detect a significant reduction in NEC. Preferably, such a study should be conducted without investigators who receive a fee for conducting the study, employees of the company or paid consultants. If such a study shows positive results, it might also reduce the price of the product, as the costs of providing infants commercial available pasteurized human milk up to discharge is at present at least USD 10,000–15,000 per child.

Pasteurization of mother's own milk for preterm infants does not reduce the incidence of late-onset sepsis

Cossey V[1,2], Vanhole C[1], Eerdekens A[1], Rayyan M[1], Fieuws S[3], Schuermans A[2]

[1]Neonatal Intensive Care Unit and [2]Department of Hospital Hygiene and Infection Control, University Hospitals Leuven and [3]Interuniversity Centre for Biostatistics and Statistical Bioinformatics, Department of Public Health, Leuven, Belgium

Neonatology 2013; 103: 170–176

Background: Human milk benefits preterm very low birth weight (VLBW) infants and may lower their risk for late-onset sepsis. Due to lack of microbiological standards, practices such as pasteurization of mother's own milk differ widely among neonatal intensive care units worldwide. Several neonatal units have a policy to pasteurize own mother's milk before administering the milk to the infants to reduce the risk of providing contaminated milk, whereas others provide unpasteurized own mother's milk. The objective of this randomized controlled trial was to investigate whether pasteurization of mother's own milk for very-low-birth-weight (VLBW) infants influences the incidence and severity of infection-related outcomes.
Methods: Infants whose mothers intended to breastfeed were randomly assigned to receive either raw or pasteurized mother's own milk. The duration of the study was from birth to 8 weeks of age or to discharge from the NICU, whichever occurred first. The primary outcome was the incidence of proven nosocomial infection.
Results: The study randomized 303 preterm infants (mean birth weight 1,276 g, mean gestational age 29 weeks). The findings of the study demonstrated that the incidence of laboratory-confirmed

sepsis was not statistically different in infants fed raw milk compared to infants who received pasteurized milk: 22/151 (0.15; CI 0.08–0.20) and 31/152 (0.20; CI 0.14–0.27), respectively (RR 0.71; 95% CI 0.43–1.17).

Conclusion: Pasteurization of mother's own milk given to VLBW infants during hospitalization in the NICU is an intervention that does not improve infection-related outcomes, such as late-onset sepsis.

Comments   Holder pasteurization is an effective method in eliminating pathogens from human milk, but has the disadvantage to reduce the immunological capacity and negatively affects the nutrient quality [4]. This study was initially powered to detect a difference in the incidence of proven nosocomial infection, but no statistical significant difference was detected. Consequently, the authors suggest that pasteurization of own mother's milk does not reduce the incidence of nosocomial infections. That is the appropriate way of concluding the results. The authors suggest that the lack of power was related to the higher rate of sepsis in their retrospective data (40%), on which they performed the power calculation, as compared to the actual incidence (17.5%). A bias in their results might be that whenever the milk of the infants in the 'raw milk' group contained specific bacteria, own mother's milk was pasteurized before administration, which happened in 16% of the infants. This might underestimate the reduction in infection incidence, and is a practice which is not frequently used around the world. In addition, the study was not blinded, although culture-proven sepsis is an outcome that is hard to influence. Despite these disadvantages, primary and several secondary outcomes tended towards slightly better outcomes in the raw milk group. No negative effects were observed by not pasteurizing own mother's milk. These results do not support the practice that own mother's milk should be pasteurized, although the final verdict is still out.

Infant Nutrition

Lactobacillus reuteri DSM 17938 for the management of infantile colic in breastfed infants: a randomized, double-blind, placebo-controlled trial

Szajewska H[1], Gyrczuk E[2], Horvath A[1]

[1]Department of Pediatrics, The Medical University of Warsaw, Warsaw, Poland; [2]Department of Family Medicine, The Medical University of Warsaw, Poland

J Pediatr 2013; 162: 257–262

Background: Infantile colic is common during the first 3–4 months of life. Depending on the definition used, colic affects 3–28% of infants, causing considerable stress and concern for parents. The pathogenesis of the condition remains elusive and many causes and/or risk factors have been suggested including the microbiota that are known to interfere with gut motor function and gas production. The objective of this study was to determine whether administration of *Lactobacillus reuteri* DSM 17938 is beneficial in breastfed infants with infantile colic.

Methods: Infants aged <5 months (n = 80) with infantile colic (crying episodes lasting ≥3 h/day and occurring at least 3 days/week within 7 days prior to enrollment) who were exclusively or predominantly (>50%) breastfed were randomly assigned to receive orally *L. reuteri* DSM 17938 [10^8 colony-forming units (CFU)] (n = 40) or identically appearing and tasting placebo (n = 40), in 5 drops, once a day, for 21 days. The primary outcome measures were the treatment success, defined as the percentage of children achieving a reduction in the daily average crying time ≥50%, and the duration of crying (minutes per day) at 7, 14, 21, and 28 days after randomization.

Results: The rate of responders to treatment was significantly higher in the probiotic group compared with the placebo group at day 7 (p = 0.026), at day 14 [relative risk (RR) 4.3; 95% CI 2.3–8.7], at day 21 [RR 2.7; 95% CI 1.85–4.1], and at day 28 [RR 2.5; 95% CI 1.8–3.75]. Throughout the study period, the median crying time was significantly reduced in the probiotic group compared with the control group. Additionally, a significant reduction in the parental perception of colic severity and an improved parental/family quality of life were found in the probiotic group compared with the placebo group. No adverse events associated with the probiotic therapy were observed.

Conclusion: The lack of effective therapy for predominately breastfed infants with infantile colic and the good safety profile of probiotics (*L. reuteri* DSM 17938) are in favor of this treatment.

Comments   Many experimental studies show that several probiotics have positive effects on mucosal immune function and have directly or indirectly anti-inflammatory properties. However, data on clinical benefits of probiotics in infancy are scarce. This study confirms the results of a study published in 2010 by Italian investigators showing that *L. reuteri* given orally at the dose of 10^8 CFU to predominantly breastfed infants improved symptoms of infantile colic with no adverse events [5]. To a lesser extent a beneficial effect on infantile colic was also noted in the control group, which may be related to the natural history of infantile colic or a placebo effect. The study also showed an improvement in parental perception of colic severity and quality of life in the group treated with the probiotic strain. It should be kept in mind that both the Italian study and the present Polish study have been performed in breastfed infants. No data are available as to whether the addition of *L. reuteri* DSM 17938 to infant formula may also improve infantile colic in formula-fed infants. Sadly, health claims related to the efficiency of *L. reuteri* DSM 17938 can be found on the labeling of infant formulae available on the market in some European countries.

Timing of the introduction of complementary feeding and risk of childhood obesity: a systematic review

Pearce J[1], Taylor MA[2], Langley-Evans SC[1]

[1]Division of Nutritional Sciences, School of Biosciences, University of Nottingham, Sutton Bonington, Loughborough, UK; [2]School of Biomedical Sciences, University of Nottingham, Queens Medical Centre, Nottingham, UK

Int J Obes (Lond) 2013 (E-pub ahead of print)

Background: In 2007, the Committee on Nutrition of the European Society for Paediatric Gastroenterology, Hepatology and Nutrition (ESPGHAN) recommended that in all infants, in consideration of their nutritional needs and developmental abilities, the complementary foods introduction should not be before 17 weeks and should not be delayed beyond 26 weeks [6]. In practice, complementary feeding is often introduced earlier than recommended. In developed countries, early introduction of complementary feeding has been associated with gastrointestinal problems, respiratory tract infections and an increased risk for allergy. The relationship to growth and body composition is unclear. The consumption of specific foods may result in the epigenetic modification of metabolic programming, or there could be a hormonal link between the duration of exclusive breastfeeding and the introduction of complementary feeding on overweight and obesity later in life. The objective of this review was to investigate the relationship between the timing of introduction of complementary feeding and overweight or obesity during childhood.

Methods: Electronic databases were searched from inception until 30 September 2012 using specified keywords. Following the application of strict inclusion/exclusion criteria, 23 studies were identified and reviewed by two independent reviewers. Data were extracted and aspects of quality were assessed.

Results: Twenty-one of the studies considered the relationship between the time at which complementary foods were introduced and childhood body mass index (BMI). Five studies found that introducing complementary foods at <3 months (2 studies), 4 months (2 studies) or 20 weeks (1 study) was associated with a higher BMI in childhood. Seven of the studies considered the association between complementary feeding and body composition but only one study reported an increase in the percentage of body fat among children given complementary foods before 15 weeks of age.

Conclusion: The timing of introduction of complementary foods has no clear association with childhood obesity, although very early introduction of solid foods ($\leq$4 months of age) may result in increased childhood BMI.

The types of food introduced during complementary feeding and risk of childhood obesity: a systematic review

Pearce J, Langley-Evans SC

Division of Nutritional Sciences, School of Biosciences, University of Nottingham, Loughborough, UK

Int J Obes (Lond) 2013; 37: 477–485

Background: The determinants of childhood overweight and obesity are multiple and complex, but infant feeding and the early diet are important contributing factors. The objective of this review was to investigate whether the type of foods given during the complementary feeding period had an impact on BMI and body composition in children aged 4–12 years.

Methods: A systematic review of the literature investigated the relationship between the types of food consumed by infants during the complementary feeding period and overweight or obesity during childhood. Electronic databases were searched from inception until June 2012. Following the application of strict inclusion/exclusion criteria, 10 studies were identified and reviewed by two independent reviewers. Studies were categorized into three groups: macronutrient intake, food type/group and adherence to dietary guidelines.

Results: In some studies, an association was found between high protein intakes at 2–12 months of age and higher BMI or body fatness in childhood. Higher BMI in childhood was associated with higher energy intake during complementary feeding. Adherence to dietary guidelines during weaning was associated with a higher lean mass, but consuming specific foods or food groups made no difference to children's BMI.

Conclusion: In very early infancy, a high energy intake, particularly dairy protein, may lead to higher BMI and higher body fatness during childhood. Further research is needed to establish this relationship. However, adherence to dietary guidelines during infancy may represent a greater likelihood of a healthy family diet, which leads to increased lean mass.

Weight change before and after the introduction of solids: results from a longitudinal birth cohort

Van Rossem L[1–3], Kiefte-de Jong JC[1,4], Looman CWN[2], Jaddoe VWV[1,4,5], Hofman A[5], Hokken-Koelega ACS[6], Mackenbach JP[2], Moll HA[4], Raat H[2]

[1]The Generation R Study Group, Erasmus MC, University Medical Center Rotterdam, Rotterdam, The Netherlands; [2]Department of Public Health, Erasmus MC, University Medical Center Rotterdam, Rotterdam, The Netherlands; [3]Julius Center for Health Sciences and Primary Care, University Medical Center Utrecht, Utrecht, The Netherlands; [4]Department of Paediatrics, Erasmus MC, University Medical Center Rotterdam, Rotterdam, The Netherlands; [5]Department of Epidemiology, Erasmus MC, University Medical Center Rotterdam, Rotterdam, The Netherlands; [6]Department of Paediatrics, Division of Endocrinology, Erasmus MC, University Medical Center Rotterdam, Rotterdam, The Netherlands

Br J Nutr 2013; 109: 370–375

Background: One mechanism underlying the higher prevalence of obesity in children is the early introduction to solids that has been described in some studies as an accelerator of infant weight gain. Intake of fatty and sugary foods has been reported to be higher at 12 months in children with early introduction to solids. Another explanation is that infant weight gain precedes the introduction of solids. Indeed, a study showed that one of the reasons for parents to introduce solids earlier than recommended is that their infant was big for their age. The objective of this study was to examine the association between the very early (0–3 months), early (between 3 and 6 months) and timely (beyond 6 months) introduction of solids and weight change in infancy and early childhood. The authors hypothesized that infants that were introduced to solids very early and early were already heavier before introduction than infants who were introduced to solids after the age of 6 months.

Methods: Data from 3,184 children were used. The association, and its direction, between the introduction of solids and weight-for-height (WFH) change between birth and 45 months of age were studied. Pregnant women were asked to participate in a birth cohort (Generation R Study) during their first antenatal visit. The timing of the introduction of solids was reported by the mother from a questionnaire at 12 months postpartum and categorized into timing of solids introduction. Anthropometric data were collected during standardized child health center visits. Repeated-measurements analyses with splines positioned according to the time of solid introduction were used to obtain estimates for WFH change before and after the introduction of solids. Analyses were adjusted for educational level, ethnicity, smoking during pregnancy, mother's BMI, breastfeeding, history of food allergy and infant's hospital admission.

Results: Relative to mothers who introduced solids early, mothers who introduced solids after the age of 6 months were more often highly educated, non-smokers, breastfeeding for at least 6 months, and had more often an infant with a history of food allergy. Before solids were introduced, weight gain was significantly higher in children introduced to solids early (z-score = 0.65; 95% CI 0.34, 0.95) than in children introduced to solids very early (z-score = 0.02; 95% CI –0.03, 0.08) and timely (z-score = 0.04; 95% CI –0.05, –0.03). Shortly after the introduction of solids, children introduced to solids very early and early showed a relative decrease in WFH. No difference was found in WFH change between the solid introduction groups after 12 months, and at that time, weight change was as expected.

Conclusion: Children introduced early to solid foods had a higher increase in WFH before the introduction of solids than children introduced timely to solids. However, no evidence was found that early introduction of solids increases WFH.

Comments   The timely introduction of complementary foods during infancy is necessary for both nutritional and developmental reasons, and to enable the transition from milk feeding to family foods [6]. The ability of breast milk or infant/follow-on formula alone to meet requirements for macro- and micronutrients becomes limited with increasing age of the infant. Furthermore, infants gradually develop the ability to chew, and start to show an interest in foods other than milk. Complementary feeding, i.e. solid foods and liquids other than breast milk or infant/follow-on formula, is associated with major changes in both macro- and micronutrient intake. In contrast to the large literature on breast and formula feeding, little attention has been paid to the complementary feeding period, the nature of the foods given, or whether this period of significant dietary change influences later health and development. The limited scientific evidence base is reflected in considerable variation in complementary feeding recommendations between countries.

The two systematic reviews and the observational study described above increase our knowledge in the complex area of complementary feeding. We are still not able to confirm whether the timing of complementary feeding or the type of foods ingested play a role in the occurrence of overweight and obesity later in childhood. However, the observational study showed that adherence to dietary guidelines may represent a greater likelihood of a healthy family diet, which in turn leads to an increased lean mass. This highlights the need for a healthy balanced diet during childhood, rather than a focus on specific foods given or not during the complementary feeding period. Studying the association between the early introduction of complementary foods and overweight and obesity later in life is a methodological challenge: (1) the association between early introduction of solids and weight gain may be related to reverse causality: infants experiencing rapid weight gain may be earlier, or later, introduced to solids; (2) there are many confounding factors that may influence the timing of complementary feeding, including educational level, socio-economic class, cultural background, smoking during pregnancy, mother's BMI, breastfeeding, history of food allergy and infant's hospital admissions. Even if the associations were adjusted for the most important confounders in the observational study, no information was available on the exclusivity of breastfeeding and on the intake of infant formula and complementary foods; (3) the age at introduction of complementary feeding is a simple exposure measure and ignores the complex dynamics of nutrition during the first 2–3 years of life; (4) the increasing prevalence of overweight and obesity is likely to be the result of a complex mixture of genetic, environmental, social, and nutritional factors. Therefore, identifying a single risk factor among so many variables is very difficult. Randomized clinical trials on complementary feeding patterns are urgently needed.

Comparison of complementary feeding strategies to meet zinc requirements of older breastfed infants

Krebs NF, Westcott JE, Culbertson DL, Sian L, Miller LV, Hambidge KM

Department of Pediatrics, Section of Nutrition, School of Medicine, University of Colorado Denver, Aurora, CO, USA

Am J Clin Nutr 2012; 96: 30–35

Background: Because zinc concentration in breast milk (HM) declines over the early months of lactation, the zinc intake of an exclusively breastfed infant also declines. The Institute of Medicine

(IoM) set the estimated average requirement for zinc dietary intake at 2.5 mg/day. To meet physiologic requirements for zinc, the infant is progressively more dependent on complementary foods (CF). Previous studies from the same group in Denver showed that zinc intake from CF, including non-zinc-fortified infant cereal was about 0.5 mg/day at 7 months, with an additional 0.5 mg/day contributed by HM [7]. Therefore, traditional complementary feeding practices for older breastfed infants would not be able to meet zinc requirements for many infants. The primary objective of this study was to compare total daily zinc absorption and zinc status in older breastfed-only infants randomly assigned at 5 months of age (while exclusively breastfed) to different complementary feeding regimens. A secondary objective was to compare biomarkers of zinc status in the feeding groups.

Methods: Exclusively breastfed 5-month-old infants (n = 45) were randomly assigned to receive commercially available pureed meats, iron- and zinc-fortified infant cereal (IZFC), or whole-grain, iron-only-fortified infant cereal (IFC) as the first and primary CF until completion of zinc metabolic studies between 9 and 10 months of age. Measurement of the fractional absorption of zinc (FAZ) in human milk and CF was performed by using a zinc stable-isotope methodology with dual isotope ratios in urine. Calculated variables included the dietary intake from duplicate diets and 4-day test weighing, the total absorbed zinc (TAZ) from FAZ × diet zinc, and the exchangeable zinc pool size (EZP) from isotope enrichment in urine.

Results: Mean daily zinc intakes were significantly greater for the meat and IZFC groups than for the IFC group (p < 0.001); only intakes in meat and IZFC groups met estimated average requirements. Mean (±SEM) TAZ amounts were 0.80 ± 0.08, 0.71 ± 0.09, and 0.52 ± 0.05 mg/day for the meat, IZFC, and IFC groups, respectively (p = 0.027). Zinc from human milk contributed <25% of TAZ for all groups. The EZP correlated with both zinc intake (r = 0.43, p < 0.01) and TAZ (r = 0.54, p < 0.001).

Conclusion: The incorporation of meats into the dietary regimen at the time of initiation of complementary feeding is well accepted and provides an intake of zinc that meets estimated dietary requirements in a well-absorbed form. Zinc-fortified commercial infant cereals provide zinc intake and daily absorbed zinc similar to that of the meat group. Zinc requirements for older breastfed-only infants are met only with the regular consumption of either meats or zinc-fortified foods.

Comments This is an important study, not only for older exclusively breastfed infants living in underprivileged parts of the world but also for those living in affluent countries. It provides information on intestinal absorption of zinc from different complementary feeding regimens. The results of the study clearly show that the daily absorbed zinc of fully breastfed infants is well below the requirements without consumption of either foods naturally high in zinc, such as meats, or micronutrient-fortified products. The mean plasma zinc concentration tended to be higher for the meat group, but the low sensitivity of this biomarker, small sample sizes in each group, and substantial variability support conclusions that plasma zinc concentrations are primarily useful for assessment of risk of zinc deficiency of populations [8]. For clinical settings, these results confirmed the value of a good diet history to judge risk of deficiency for older infants and toddlers who are predominantly breastfed. The results of this study also support complementary feeding recommendations by the WHO for settings with low resources where deficiencies of zinc and iron in infants and young children toddlers are widespread.

Timing of the introduction of complementary foods in infancy: a randomized controlled trial

Jonsdottir OH[1], Thorsdottir I[1], Hibberd PL[2], Fewtrell MS[3], Wells JC[3], Palsson GI[4], Lucas A[3], Gunnlaugsson G[5], Kleinman RE[6]

[1]Unit for Nutrition Research, Landspitali, The National University Hospital of Iceland and Faculty of Food Science and Nutrition, University of Iceland, Reykjavik, Iceland; [2]Division of Global Health, Massachusetts General Hospital for Children, Harvard Medical School, Boston, MA, USA; [3]Childhood Nutrition Research Centre, University College London Institute of Child Health, London, UK; [4]Children's Hospital, Landspitali, The National University Hospital of Iceland; [5]Directorate of Health and Reykjavik University, Reykjavik, Iceland; [6]Department of Pediatrics, Massachusetts General Hospital for Children, Harvard Medical School, Boston, MA, USA

Pediatrics 2012; 130: 1038–1045

Background: In 2001, WHO changed the recommended duration of exclusive breastfeeding from the first 4–6 months to the first 6 months of life [9]. WHO stated that 'the available evidence demonstrates no apparent evident risks in recommending, as a general policy, exclusive breastfeeding for the first 6 months of life in both developing and developed country settings'. The principle reason for this change was to provide optimal nutrition to young infants in low-resource countries where available water and complementary foods may be nutritionally inadequate or contaminated. However, there is still some controversy as to whether the iron intake of infants exclusively breastfed for 6 months in these low-income countries is sufficient to cover their needs at the end of the first semester of life. In high-income countries, no data are available on the iron status after 4 or 6 months of exclusive breast-feeding. One systematic review of the optimal age for the introduction of complementary foods concluded that there was inadequate evidence in high-income countries to increase the duration of exclusive breastfeeding from 4 to 6 months of age. WHO has requested randomized controlled trials to be done to guide policy decisions in this regard. The objective of the study was to examine the optimal duration of exclusive breastfeeding concerning the iron status and growth rate of infants in Iceland.
Methods: In this randomized, controlled trial, healthy term ($\geq$37 weeks) singleton infants (n = 119) were randomly assigned to receive either complementary foods in addition to breast milk from the age of 4 months (CF) or to exclusive breastfeeding for 6 months (EBF). Data were collected regarding diet by 3-day weighed food records, iron status and growth.
Results: Infants in the CF group had higher mean serum ferritin (SF) levels at 6 months (70.0 ± 73.3 vs. 44.0 ± 53.8 µg/l, p = 0.02), which remained significant when adjusted for baseline characteristics. However, there was no difference between groups in the prevalence of iron deficiency anemia (Hb <10.5 g/l, MCV <74 fl, SF <12 g/l), iron deficiency (MCV <74 fl, SF <12 µg/l), or iron depletion (SF <12 µg/l). Infants in both groups grew at the same rate between 4 and 6 months of age. Mean energy intake from complementary foods at 5 months was 8.8 kcal/kg/day, which is approximately 10% of the average daily energy requirements for infants 6–11 months of age. The mean daily intake of iron from complementary foods was 0.6 mg, which is 8% of an infant's average daily iron requirements at age 6–11 months.
Conclusion: In a high-income country, infants who receive a small amount of complementary food in addition to breast milk from 4 months of age had higher iron stores at 6 months compared with those exclusively breastfed for 6 months. However, no effect was found on the growth rate between 4 and 6 months.

Comments This important study is the first one to examine the effects of exclusive breastfeeding for 4 vs. 6 months on iron status and growth in a high-income study. With respect to growth, the study confirms the conclusion of the systematic review which was the basis for the WHO recommendation regarding the optimal duration of exclusive breastfeeding. Whereas infants in the CF group had higher iron stores at 6 months compared with those in the EBF group, both groups had adequate stores as determined by SF levels and no significant differences were seen between groups in the prevalence of iron deficiency with or without anemia. Taking into account these results it is very unlikely that an infant exclusively breastfed for 6 months from a healthy mother in a high-income country will present iron deficiency/iron deficiency anemia or an impaired growth. Nevertheless, the growth pattern should be closely monitored using the WHO Child Growth Standards published in 2006 [10].

Breastfeeding duration: influence on taste acceptance over the first year of life

Schwartz C[1-3], Chabanet C[1-3], Laval C[1-3], Issanchou S[1-3], Nicklaus S[1-3]

[1]INRA, UMR1324 Center for Taste and Feeding Behaviour, Dijon, France; [2]CNRS, UMR6265, Center for Taste and Feeding Behaviour, Dijon, France; [3]University of Burgundy, Center for Taste and Feeding Behaviour, Dijon, France

Br J Nutr 2013; 109: 1154–1161

Background: Among early feeding experiences, those related to milk feeding, whether it is breastfeeding or formula feeding, can have important impact on taste acceptance, which is one of the major determinants of food consumption in children. Compared with exposure to formula, exposure to maternal milk may result in sensory difference in terms of aroma and taste. Concerning aroma, some volatile compounds from the foods ingested by the mother are likely to be transmitted into her milk. Breast milk may bear a distinct flavor component which is likely to have an impact on infant behavior at the age of complementary feeding, as shown in several studies. Concerning taste, breast milk contains some compounds which bear a taste, such as lactose (sweet taste), glutamate (umami taste), Na (salty taste) and urea (bitter taste). Their concentration in breast milk differs from that in infant formula: the concentration of glutamate may be up to 14-fold higher and the concentration of Na is 2- to 4-fold lower. The impact of breastfeeding on later taste acceptance has been rarely assessed. The objective of this study was to examine the impact of exclusive breastfeeding duration (DEB) on the acceptance of sweet, salty, sour, bitter and umami taste solutions at 6 and 12 months.

Methods: Participating mothers were recruited before the last trimester of pregnancy. Data were reported for 122 infants (62 males), with a birth weight of 3.31 (SD 0.51) kg and a birth length of 50.0 (SD 2.4) cm. Mothers recorded the DEB. Acceptance of solutions of each of the five basic tastes relative to water was evaluated at 6 and 12 months by the ingestion ratio (IR) [11]. The IR of a taste was defined as the ingested volume of this taste solution relative to the sum of the ingested volumes of this taste solution and of water. This IR is interpreted as follows: ratio at 0.5 indicates indifference to the taste solution; ratio >0.5 indicates a preference for the taste solution over water; ratio <0.5 indicates a rejection of the taste solution over water. Kendall correlations were calculated between the DEB and the IR.

Results: Only 16% of infants completed at least 6 months of exclusive breastfeeding; 79% had begun complementary feeding by 6 months. At 6 months, infants preferred sweet, salty and umami solutions over water and were indifferent to sour and bitter solutions. The longer an infant was breastfed, the more the umami solution was accepted at 6 months (p = 0.02). At 12 months, infants preferred sweet and salty solutions over water and were indifferent to sour, bitter and umami solutions. The relationship between the DEB and acceptance of the umami solution was no more observed at 12 months. No relationship was observed between the DEB and sweet, salty, sour and bitter taste acceptance at 6 or 12 months.

Conclusion: This study highlights the role of exclusive breastfeeding in the establishment of taste acceptance, with a positive impact of longer breastfeeding duration on umami taste acceptance at 6 months, maybe related to the higher glutamate content of human milk compared with formula milk. It suggests that prolonged breastfeeding could also be associated with an impact on sensory preference at the beginning of complementary feeding.

Comments   As suggested by the authors, the observed association between the DEB and umami taste preference at 6 months, studied using monosodium glutamate, is likely to be related to the effect of exposure to glutamate in breast milk. The interpretation of the results is somewhat limited by the fact that breast milk was neither analyzed for taste compound composition, nor evaluated by a sensory panel to characterize its perceived taste. The impact of exclusive breastfeeding on umami taste acceptance is transient. It was observed at an age close to the beginning of complementary feeding and could favor the initial acceptance of umami-tasting foods. This could constitute a 'taste bridge' effect, in the same way that a 'flavor bridge' effect was previously described by Mennella et al. [12] regarding flavor transition from breast milk to a solid diet. Concerning salty taste, the results of Schwartz et al. did not confirm previous findings. A specific limitation to any study on breastfeeding is that it is not possible to carry out interventional studies randomizing breastfeeding. Rate and duration of breastfeeding may vary according to several factors, in particular the mother's social status.

Even with some methodological limitations, this important paper adds more knowledge to the fascinating area of the sensory and behavioral consequences of very early feeding on feeding behavior and feeding patterns later in life. Research in the field of complementary feeding should be encouraged by governments, official bodies and research agencies and not only by the industry.

References

1 Lucas A: Programming by early nutrition: an experimental approach. J Nutr 1998;128:401S–406S.
2 ESPGHAN Committee on Nutrition, Agostoni C, Braegger C, Decsi T, Kolacek S, Koletzko B, Michaelsen KF, Mihatsch W, Moreno LA, Puntis J, Shamir R, Szajewska H, Turck D, van Goudoever J: Breast feeding: a position paper by the ESPGHAN Committee on Nutrition. J Pediatr Gastroenterol Nutr 2009;49:112–125.
3 Sullivan S, Schanler RJ, Kim JH, Patel AL, Trawöger R, Kiechl-Kohlendorfer U, Chan GM, Blanco CL, Abrams S, Cotten CM, Laroia N, Ehrenkranz RA, Dudell G, Cristofalo EA, Meier P, Lee ML, Rechtman DJ, Lucas A: An exclusively human milk-based diet is associated with a lower rate of necrotising enterocolitis than a diet of human milk and bovine milk-based products. J Pediatr 2010;156:562–567.
4 ESPGHAN Committee on Nutrition and Invited Experts, Arslanoglu S, Braegger C, Campoy C, Colomb V, Corpeleijn W, Decsi T, Domellof M, Fewtrell M, Mihatsch W, Moro G, Shamir R, Turck D, van Goudoever J: Donor human milk for preterm infants: current evidence and research directions. A comment by the ESPGHAN Committee on Nutrition. J Pediatr Gastroenterol Nutrition (in press).
5 Savino F, Cordisco L, Tarasco V, Palumeri E, Calabrese R, Oggero R, Roos S, Matteuzzi D: *Lactobacillus reuteri* DSM 17938 in infantile colic: a randomized, double-blind, placebo-controlled trial. Pediatrics 2010;126:e526.

6 ESPGHAN Committee on Nutrition, Agostoni C, Decsi T, Fewtrell M, Goulet O, Kolacek S, Koletzko B, Michaelsen KF, Moreno L, Puntis J, Rigo J, Shamir R, Szajewska H, Turck D, van Goudoever J: Complementary feeding: a commentary by the ESPGHAN Committee on Nutrition. J Pediatr Gastroenterol Nutr 2008;46:99–110.

7 Krebs NF, Reidinger CJ, Robertson AD, Hambidge KM: Growth and intakes of energy and zinc in infants fed human milk. J Pediatr 1994;124:32–39.

8 De Benoist B, Darnton-Hill I, Davidsson L, Fontaine O, Hotz C: Conclusions of the joint WHO/UNICEF/IAEA/IZiNCG interagency meeting on zinc status indicators. Food Nutr Bull 2007;28:S480–S484.

9 World Health Organization: The Optimal Duration of Exclusive Breastfeeding: Report of an Expert Consultation. Geneva, WHO, 2001. Available at: http://www.who.int/nutrition/publications/optimal_duration_of_exc_bfeeding_report_eng.pdf (accessed September 26, 2013).

10 Turck D, Michaelsen KF, Shamir R, Braegger C, Campoy C, Colomb V, et al, on behalf of the ESPGHAN Committee on Nutrition: World Health Organization 2006 Child Growth Standards and 2007 Growth References Charts: a discussion paper by the Committee on Nutrition of the European Society for Paediatric Gastroenterology, Hepatology and Nutrition. J Pediatr Gastroenterol Nutr 2013;57:258–264.

11 Schwartz C, Issanchou S, Nicklaus S: Developmental changes in the acceptance of the five basic tastes in the first year of life. Br J Nutr 2009;102:1375–1385.

12 Mennella JA, Griffin CE, Beauchamp GK: Flavor programming during infancy. Pediatrics 2004;113:840–845.

Koletzko B, Shamir R, Turck D, Phillip M (eds): Nutrition and Growth: Yearbook 2014.
World Rev Nutr Diet. Basel, Karger, 2014, vol 109, pp 36–53 (DOI: 10.1159/000356107)

Cognition

Holly R. Hull and Susan E. Carlson

Department of Dietetics and Nutrition at the University of Kansas Medical Center, Kansas City, KS, USA

This chapter in the *Yearbook on Nutrition and Growth* summarizes the articles that have been published in the area of cognition and nutrition. Articles were included if published (including E-pub ahead of press) between the dates July 1, 2012 and June 30, 2013. All studies were human observational or clinical trials. The topics or nutrients explored in the articles naturally fell into one of three categories: feeding studies (breastfeeding and school feeding), long-chain polyunsaturated fatty acids supplementation (LCPUFA) and micronutrients (methyl donors and iodine, iron and vitamin A). Comments are included following the summaries of papers within each category.

Feeding Studies: Infant Feeding

Role of breastfeeding in childhood cognitive development: a propensity score matching analysis

Boutwell BB[1], Beaver KM[3], Barnes JC[2]

[1]College of Criminal Justice, Sam Houston State University, Huntsville, TX, USA; [2]University of Texas at Dallas, Richardson, TX, USA; [3]College of Criminology and Criminal Justice, Florida State University, Tallahassee, FL, USA

J Paediatr Child Health 2012; 48: 840–845

Background: Children that have been breastfed score higher on IQ tests when compared to children who were formula-fed. Some suggest the beneficial effect from breastfeeding is an artifact of the situation. Women who decide to breastfeed differ from women who decide to use formula. The purpose was to explore the association between breastfeeding and offspring cognitive scores to determine if the relationship is direct or due to confounding variables.

Methods: A novel statistical analysis, propensity score matching (PSM), was used to analyze data from the Early Childhood Longitudinal Study, Birth Cohort. PSM approximates a randomized research design using observational data by matching data from two groups. Children who were breastfed were matched on several different potentially confounding variables to children who were fed commercial infant formula. A total of 10,700 mother-child pairs were used in this analysis. The Bayley Short Form-Research Edition (BSF-R) was used to assess cognitive function when the offspring were 2 years old.

Results: Initially, nine of the twelve potential confounding variables differed between groups. After matching, group differences remained for only one variable (a small difference in birth weight). After reducing differences between groups for confounding variables, the effect of breastfeeding on cognitive scores was calculated. Prior to matching, the association between breastfeeding and cognition was significant (mean difference 3.20; $p \leq 0.05$). After matching, the significance remained but was attenuated by 40% (mean difference 1.92; $p \leq 0.05$).

Conclusion: Using PSM, the beneficial effect of breastfeeding on offspring cognition is supported. Further research is needed to understand the pathways for this effect.

Infant feeding: the effects of scheduling vs. on-demand feeding on mothers' wellbeing and children's cognitive development

Iacovou M[1], Sevilla A[2]

[1]Institute for Social and Economic Research, University of Essex, Colchester, UK; [2]Department of Economics and Centre for Time Use Research, University of Oxford, Oxford, UK

Eur J Public Health 2012; 23: 13–19

Background: Two predominate infant feeding styles are feeding on demand or feeding to a schedule. Proponents of feeding to a schedule suggest this feeding style leads to a happier baby that sleeps through the night earlier, lowers the level of parental stress and provides neurocognitive developmental advantages. The purpose was to compare children's long-term cognitive development and academic performance based on maternal self-identified infant feeding style.

Methods: Participants were part of the Avon Longitudinal Study of Parents and Children. A total of 10,419 mother-child pairs were grouped as 'on demand' or 'scheduled' feeders for this analysis based on mothers' answers at 4 weeks post-partum to the questions: '*Is your baby fed on a regular schedule?*' At 8 years of age, cognitive development was assessed by IQ tests and academic performance scores were determined with the Standard Attainment Test (SAT). The SAT is standardized for use in children from the age of 5 to 14 years.

Results: After controlling for multiple confounding variables, infants fed to a schedule had lower SAT scores at all ages and lower IQ scores (–4 points) at 8 years of age compared to those fed on demand.

Conclusion: Differences were found between groups based on maternal identified feeding style. Children fed on demand during infancy had higher cognitive and academic performance scores when compared to children fed to a schedule during infancy. Further testing controlling infant feeding style is needed to explore these results.

Comments The study of Boutwell et al. asks an old question: Is higher IQ consistently observed in breastfed compared to formula-fed infants due to the composition of human milk or some other environmental benefit associated with feeding choice. Unlike past studies, they used a novel statistical approach (propensity score matching) to examine a very large US birth cohort of 10,700 mother-child pairs. They observed an effect on the Bayley Short Form that was 3.2 points higher in breastfed infants before matching the groups for differences in potentially confounding variables. This is similar to a 4-point advantage that has been found quite consistently with the Bayley Scales of Infant Development Mental Developmental Index (BSID MDI). After matching for all but one potentially confounding variable, the difference between the groups became quite small (1.92 points) but was still statistically significant. All studies that attempt to control for potentially influential variables have the limitation that they may have failed to control for an important unknown variable that could account for this small difference. Moreover, commercial infant formulas continue to be modified to be more similar to human milk in composition and functionality. For example, changes in formula after this cohort completed the first year of life include the addition of DHA and ARA to US formulas (2002) and the inclusion of pre- and probiotics in some formulas (also see the section on LCPUFA for evidence of cognitive benefit of formula LCPUFA supplementation). As a result, it is unlikely that this question will have a definitive answer anytime soon.

Iacovou and Sevilla looked at the relationship between on-demand vs. scheduled feeding in infancy on childhood IQ and academic performance. They found both were higher in 8-year-old children who were fed on demand. We are inclined to read this as evidence that encouraging infant self-regulation can produce important benefits for subsequent child development. As far as we know, this is the first study to evaluate self-regulation in relation to cognitive function or academic performance. We expect it will lead to many more studies on this subject.

Feeding Studies: School Feeding Studies

Refined carbohydrate intake in relation to non-verbal intelligence among Tehrani schoolchildren

Abargouei AS[1,2], Kalantari N[3], Omidvar N[3], Rashidkhani B[3], Rad AH[4], Ebrahimi AA[4], Khosravi-Boroujeni H[1], Esmaillzadeh A[1,2]

[1]Food Security Research Center, Isfahan University of Medical Sciences, Isfahan, Islamic Republic of Iran; [2]Department of Community Nutrition, School of Nutrition and Food Science, Isfahan University of Medical Sciences, Islamic Republic of Iran; [3]Department of Community Nutrition, Faculty of Nutrition and Food Technology, Shahid Beheshti University of Medical Sciences, Teheran, Islamic Republic of Iran; [4]National Nutrition and Food Technology Institute, Shahid Beheshti University of Medical Sciences, Teheran, Islamic Republic of Iran

Public Health Nutr 2012; 15: 1925–1931

Background: Adequate micronutrient consumption is known to be essential for cognitive development. Carbohydrate and in particular glucose and the glycemic index are thought to also influence cognitive function but few studies exist. The purpose of the study was to examine the relationship between refined carbohydrate intake and intelligence quotient (IQ) in schoolchildren.

Methods: 245 children aged 6–7 years from 129 elementary schools in Tehran, Iran, participated. Intelligence was measured by Raven's Colorful Progressive Matrices and a food frequency questionnaire assessed dietary intake of refined carbohydrates in the last year.

Results: Children were divided into tertiles based on the amount of refined carbohydrate consumed. After controlling for potential confounding variables, difference in IQ scores among the tertiles of refined carbohydrate intake were not found, however non-verbal IQ scores and refined carbohydrate intake were inversely related. After adjusting for all potential confounding variables, the negative relationship remained (β = –8.495; p = 0.038).

Conclusion: These data suggest a negative relationship between refined carbohydrate intake and non-verbal intelligence scores in young schoolchildren from Tehran, Iran. Further studies controlling refined carbohydrate intake and assessing intelligence are needed to confirm these findings.

The effect of beverages varying in glycemic load on postprandial glucose responses, appetite and cognition in 10- to 12-year-old schoolchildren

Brindal E[1], Baird D[1], Slater A[2], Danthiir V[1], Wilson C[3], Bowen J[1], Noakes M[1]

[1]CSIRO Food and Nutritional Sciences, Adelaide, SA, Australia; [2]Flinders University, Adelaide, SA, Australia; [3]Cancer Council South Australia and Flinders Centre for Cancer Prevention and Control, Flinders University, Adelaide, SA, Australia

Br J Nutr 2013; 110: 529–537

Background: Consumption of breakfast in children is related to higher cognitive performance. A proposed underlying mechanism conferring the beneficial effect is postconsumption stabilized glucose levels. The impact of breakfast varying in glycemic load (GL) on cognition is unknown. The purpose was to assess the effect of a breakfast drink with varying levels of carbohydrate relative to fat and protein on cognitive function.

Methods: 40 children aged 10–12 years participated in this double-blind, randomized, three-way repeated measures crossover design study. Three isoenergetic drinks were given: a glucose beverage (glycemic index (GI) 100, GL 65), a full milk beverage (GI 27, GL 5) and a half milk/glucose beverage (GI 84, GL 35). For the next 3 h, cognition was tested hourly. Six cognitive constructs were assessed: speed of processing, attention switching, perceptual speed, short-term and working memory, and inspection time. Blood glucose levels were monitored throughout with a Continuous Glucose Monitoring System (CGMS).

Results: Blood glucose AUC differed between conditions as expected (p < 0.001). No main effects were found for test drink on any of the cognitive assessments. A significant interaction was detected between gender and drink GL for short-term memory. A greater number of words were recalled by girls when they consumed either milk containing beverage (0.7–0.8 words) compared to the glucose beverage (0.5 words; p ≤ 0.014).

Conclusion: No effect on cognitive performance was found when GL was varied in a breakfast drink for the group as a whole, however girls had higher short-term memory scores after consuming the two protein-containing beverages compared to glucose alone.

Effects of lunch on children's short-term cognitive functioning: a randomized crossover study

Muller K[1], Libuda L[1], Gawehn N[2], Drossard C[1,4], Bolzenius K[1], Kunz C[3], Kersting M[1]

[1]Application-Oriented Research, Research Institute of Child Nutrition (FKE), Dortmund, Germany; [2]University of Applied Health Sciences, Bochum, Germany; [3]Institute of Nutritional Science, Justus Liebig University Giessen, Giessen, Germany

Eur J Clin Nutr 2013; 67: 185–189

Background: Skipping breakfast is related to poorer cognitive performance in schoolchildren though the impact of skipping lunch on cognitive performance has only been investigated in adults. European schools commonly last for a full day, however students do not consistently consume lunch. The purpose of this study was to investigate the effect of consuming lunch on cognitive performance.

Methods: 105 sixth grade children participated in this randomized, crossover controlled trial. The study took place at an all-day school in Germany that served warm lunches. There were 2 test days separated by 1 week. On 1e day, children were tested after skipping lunch and another after having lunch. Classes were randomized to test order. Cognitive assessment occurred immediately following the lunch break. The computerized test battery of the Vienna Test System and its subtests assessed alertness, immediate block span (visuospatial performance) and selective attention.

Results: After adjustment for multiple testing, no differences between groups were found for any of the cognitive tests.

Conclusion: Skipping lunch had no adverse effect on a short-term measure of cognitive performance in sixth grade children. Further research is needed to verify these results and explore the underlying mechanisms.

Early-stage primary schoolchildren attending school in the Malawian school feeding program (SFP) have better reversal learning and lean muscle mass growth than those attending a non-SFP school

Nikhoma OWW[1,2], Duffy ME[2], Cory-Slechta DA[3], Davidson PW[3], McSorley EM[2], Strain JJ[2], O'Brien GM[2]

[1]University of Malawi, Chancellor College, Zomba, Malawi; [2]University of Ulster, School Biomedical Sciences, Northern Ireland Centre for Food and Health, Coleraine, UK; [3]University of Rochester, School of Medicine and Dentistry, Rochester, NY, USA

J Nutr 2013; 143: 1324–1330

Background: School feeding programs (SFP) have been adopted in developing countries as a way to improve children's nutrition, cognitive development and academic performance. Conflicting evidence exists regarding the effectiveness of SFP. The purpose was to assess cognition in children attending a school that was receiving additional nutrition through the SFP in Malawi, Southern Africa.

Methods: Children aged 6–8 years in two rural public primary schools (one SFP school and one non-SFP school) were followed for 1 year. A total of 226 children completed baseline and follow-up testing. Children in the SFP received a daily ration of corn-soy porridge while children in the non-SFP did not. The Cambridge Neurological Test Automated Battery (CAN-TAB) was used to assess the following domains of cognition related to behavior: learning, set-shifting, memory and attention and 3 subtests to assess brain cognitive domains including memory, reversal learning and attention.

Results: A significant improvement in reversal learning was observed in the SFP children between baseline and follow-up testing. The group had a greater reduction in the number of intra-extra pre-dimensional shift errors compared to the non-SFP group (p = 0.02).

Conclusion: Results suggest the additional nutrition provided by SFP is beneficial for short-term cognitive development in children from underdeveloped countries who have poor access to food.

Comments Two studies published this year looked at carbohydrate quality and cognition in school-children. Abargouei et al. measured intelligence in 6- to 7-year-old Iranian children who were divided into tertiles based on their refined carbohydrate intake. While they did not find any relationship between refined carbohydrate intake and overall IQ, intake was inversely related to non-verbal intelligence scores even after adjusting for potentially confounding variables. More targeted tests of cognitive function might have been a better choice for outcome than IQ, which should be quite stable at this age. Brindal et al. provided 10- to 12-year-old Australian children isocaloric breakfasts that varied in glucose and milk content. While they found no main effects on any of the cognitive assessments, girls performed better on a test for short-term memory (word recall) if they consumed either a milk-containing beverage compared to a beverage that contained only glucose. German sixth grade children participated in a randomized, crossover controlled study of the relationship between lunch consumption and tests to assess alertness, visuospatial performance and selective attention. After adjusting for multiple testing, no differences were found between children's performance when they ate lunch compared to when they did not. In contrast, Malawian children (6–8 years of age) performed better on the CAN-TAB (which assesses learning, memory and attention, and reversal learning and attention) when given a daily ration of a corn-soy porridge. Both of these studies provided a meal to children who otherwise would likely have been hungry. Both measured a similar cognitive behavior. The difference in results could be due to differences in energy reserves between the two populations or to differences in age, with younger children being more susceptible to hunger.

Long-Chain Polyunsaturated Fatty Acid Studies

Long-term effects of LCPUFA supplementation on childhood cognitive outcomes

Colombo J[1], Carlson SE[2], Cheatham CL[2], Shaddy DJ[2], Kerling EH[2], Thodosoff JM[2], Gustafson KM[3], Brez C[1]

[1]Schiefelbusch Life Span Institute and Department of Psychology, University of Kansas, Kansas City, KS, USA; [2]Department of Dietetics and Nutrition, University of Kansas Medical Center, Kansas City, KS, USA; [3]Hoglund Brain Imaging Center, University of Kansas Medical Center, Kansas City, KS, USA

Am J Clin Nutr 2013; 98: 403–412

Background: Long-chain polyunsaturated fatty acids (LCPUFA) are thought to play a role in neuro-cognitive development during infancy. Data vary regarding whether LCPUFA supplementation during infancy results in a positive neurocognitive effect during early childhood. This study reported results for age-appropriate neurocognitive assessment at 6-month intervals between 18 months and 6 years of age in children supplemented with infant formula for 12 months with varying doses of DHA.

Methods: 81 children participated in the randomized, double-blind, DHA dose-response controlled trial. Newborn term infants were randomized to one of four groups varying in DHA (0.32, 0.64 and 0.96% of total fatty acids) with 0.64% arachidonic acid (ARA) or control (0% DHA and ARA). Cognitive testing occurred at 18 months of age and every 6 months thereafter until 6 years of age. The cognitive assessments performed at each time point varied and were age-appropriate.
Results: No differences between groups were found at 18 months for infant development or early communication skills (MCDI) or BSID MDI or at any time point for tasks of spatial memory, simple inhibition or advanced problem-solving. The middle dose groups (0.32 and 0.64%) had significantly increased rule-learning and inhibition task scores at 4 and 5 years on the Dimensional Change Card Sort (DCCS) task and had greater vocabulary scores at age 5 years (PPVT) compared to the control group. The highest 2 doses (0.64 and 0.96%) had higher scores than the control group on the Stroop test across the ages of 3–5 years. The Stroop tested ability to follow a rule that ran counter to an automatic response. All of these findings were significant when supplemented groups were combined and compared to control. Advantages were found for the combined DHA-supplemented groups compared to control infants on several cognitive tests to 5 years of age as well as on full-scale and verbal IQ at 6 years of age.
Conclusion: DHA and AA supplementation in infancy increased cognitive scores to age 6. These results suggest that increasing DHA status early in development benefits cognitive development at school age.

Effects of long-chain polyunsaturated fatty acid supplementation of infant formula on cognition and behavior at 9 years of age

De Jong C[1], Kikkert HK[1], Fidler V[2], Hadders-Algra M[1]

[1]Department of Paediatrics, Institute of Developmental Neurology, University Medical Center Groningen, Groningen, The Netherlands; [2]Department of Epidemiology, University Medical Center Groningen, Groningen, The Netherlands

Dev Med Child Neurol 2012; 54: 1102–1108

Background: Long-chain polyunsaturated fatty acids (LCPUFA) are thought to be important for early cognitive development, but few studies have assessed neurocognitive development at any time in childhood. This study reported cognitive and behavioral findings in 9-year-olds that received formula supplemented with LCPUFA in infancy and examined the potential confounding effect of perinatal maternal smoking.
Methods: The design was a double-blind, randomized control trial. 474 healthy term infants were recruited at birth. Three groups were followed for 9 years: the control group (n = 169) received standard formula (SF), the intervention group (EF; n = 145) received DHA- and AA-enriched formula, and the third group was fed human milk (BF; n = 160). Supplementation duration was birth to 2 months. Mothers reported smoking habits during pregnancy. The Wechsler Abbreviated Scale of Intelligence was administered at 9 years of age. Scores were reported as full IQ (FIQ) and those scores that comprised FIQ: verbal IQ (VIQ) and performance IQ (PIQ). A Developmental Neuropsychological Assessment (NEPSY) was used to assess executive function and memory and learning.
Results: Breastfeeding provided benefits regardless of maternal smoking: children exposed in utero to smoking who were BF had greater FIQ and learning and memory scores (p < 0.05) when compared to SF. Offspring exposed to smoking and given EF or BF also had higher VIQ scores when compared to the SF group (p < 0.05). Among non-smoking pregnancies, children who were BF had greater FIQ (p = 0.026) and learning and memory scores (p = 0.012) compared to EF. Subset IQ scores varied by infant nutrition and smoking exposure.

Conclusion: Breastfeeding continues to provide benefits for neurocognitive and behavioral development at 9 years of age. The beneficial effect of LCPUFA enrichment was inconsistent and influenced by maternal smoking.

Effects of high-dose fish oil supplementation during early infancy on neurodevelopment and language: a randomized controlled trial

Meldrum SJ[1,2], D'Vaz N[1], Simmer K[1,2], Dunstan JA[1], Hird K[1,3], Prescott SL[1]

[1]School of Paediatrics and Child Health, University of Western Australia, Crawley, WA, Australia;
[2]School of Women's and Infants Health, University of Western Australia, Crawley, WA, Australia;
[3]Faculty of Medicine, Notre Dame University, Freemantle, WA, Australia

Br J Nutr 2012; 108: 1443–1454

Background: Supplementation of long-chain polyunsaturated fatty acids (LCPUFA) during pregnancy and infancy is proposed to have beneficial effects on offspring neurocognitive development. Supplementation studies have found mixed results regarding benefits of LCPUFA supplementation on infant neurocognitive function. This study directly supplemented infants for the first 6 months of life to determine if supplementation improved global infant neurodevelopment and early communication.
Methods: A randomized, double-blind, placebo-controlled trial recruited 420 healthy term infants. The intervention group (n = 218) received DHA-enriched fish oil (250 mg DHA/day and 60 mg EPA/day) and the placebo group (n = 202) received olive oil. At 12 and 18 months, language was assessed by the MacArthur-Bates Communicative Development Inventory (MCDI) and at 18 months the Bayley Scales of Infant and Toddler Development (BSID-III) and the Achenbach Child Behavior Checklist (CBCL) were assessed. The MCDI was repeated at 18 months.
Results: Cord blood fatty acids were analyzed and the results confirmed that both groups had a similar DHA status at birth. At the end of the intervention, the intervention group had greater erythrocyte fatty acid (FA) measured DHA and EPA and lower AA levels (p < 0.05) when compared to the placebo group. No group differences were found for the BSID-III though in a subset analysis of the MCDI, differences were found at 12 and 18 months for language assessments as reflected by higher gesture scores (p < 0.05) in the intervention group.
Conclusion: Global infant neurodevelopment was not improved by early postnatal supplementation of a high dose of LCPUFA. Subset analysis did find greater language skill development in the supplemented group.

Long-chain PUFA supplementation in rural African infants: a randomized controlled trial of effects on gut integrity, growth and cognitive development

Van der Merwe LF[1,3], Moore SE[1,3], Fulford AJ[1,3], Halliday KE[2], Drammeh S[3], Young S[4], Prentice AM[1,3]

[1]Medical Research Council International Nutrition Group, London School of Hygiene and Tropical Medicine, London, UK; [2]Faculty of Infectious and Tropical Disease, London School of Hygiene and Tropical Medicine, London, UK; [3]MRC Keneba, Keneba, The Gambia; [4]Medical Research Council Human Nutrition Research, Elsie Widdowson Laboratory, Cambridge, UK

Am J Clin Nutr 2013; 97: 45–57

Background: Harsh environmental conditions experienced in third world countries can influence gut integrity causing malabsorption leading to poor growth and development in newborns. Long-chain polyunsaturated fatty acid (LCPUFA) supplements are associated with a reduction in inflammation and higher neurocognitive development. No study has investigated if LCPUFA can reduce gastrointestinal inflammation and improve neurocognitive development in rural Gambian infants.

Methods: 183 breastfed infants participated in the randomized, double-blind controlled trial. An LCPUFA (DHA and EPA) supplement was given as a capsule of fish oil (2 ml) (200 mg DHA/day and 300 mg EPA/day; n = 92) to infants daily from 3 to 9 months. The control group (CON; n = 91) received olive oil (2 ml). Anthropometrics were used to assess growth and the lactulose:mannitol ratio was used as a marker of gut integrity. Cognitive development was assessed at 12 months using the Willatts' Infant Planning Test and a single object task attention assessment.

Results: Supplementation increased the percentage of DHA and EPA in plasma total lipids (p < 0.001). At 9 and 12 months, mid upper arm circumference and triceps skinfold was greater in the FO group compared to the CON though no differences in weight-for-age or weight-for-length were detected. No differences between groups were found for markers of inflammation, gut integrity or neurocognitive development.

Conclusion: Supplementation increased infant n–3 LCPUFA status in Gambian infants. Anthropometric differences were found for markers of adiposity, however no differences were found for markers of inflammation, gut integrity or neurocognitive development.

Comments Four papers published this year evaluated the effects of supplementing infants with long-chain polyunsaturated omega-3 fatty acids. Three of these involved cognitive tests done after supplementation was discontinued for at least 6 months and as long as 9 years. All three were conducted in developed countries. De Jong et al. studied 9-year-old children who had been fed either standard formula or DHA- and ARA-enriched formula for the first 2 months of life. A third group received human milk. Meldrum et al. studied 12- and 18-month-old children who took a DHA-enriched fish oil capsule or a placebo group that took an olive oil capsule for the first 6 months of life. Colombo et al. studied cognitive outcomes in children from 18 months to 6 years of life at 6-month intervals who had received formulas with one of four concentrations of DHA during the first 12 months of life – 0, 0.32, 0.64 and 0.96% DHA of total dietary fatty acid (the DHA-containing formulas also provided 0.64% ARA).

Full-scale (FIQ) and verbal IQ (VIQ) were measured at school age by both de Jong et al. and Colombo et al. Children supplemented with DHA and ARA had higher FIQ and VIQ at 6 years in the latter study. VIQ was significantly higher in the de Jong et al. study with formula containing DHA and ARA compared to standard formula only among offspring of women who smoked. A major difference between these studies was the duration of feeding of supplemented formula in infancy. Both suggest benefits to verbal IQ at school age. Other targeted cognitive outcomes found to be higher in DHA- and ARA-supplemented children by Colombo et al. included higher scores on the PPVT at 5 years and on tests that required the child to follow a rule counter to an automatic response (Stroop) or inhibit a learned rule (DCCS). An earlier report from this cohort of children found higher sustained attention at 9 months of age in the combined supplemented groups compared to the control group.

In agreement with Meldrum et al., Colombo et al. found no effect of DHA and ARA in infant formula on the MCDI and the BSID-III at 18 months of age. Both studies concluded that global toddler neurodevelopment was not improved by early postnatal supplementation. Meldrum et al. did find a suggestion that early communication (based on gestures) was enhanced by fish oil supplementation. It would be interesting to see more targeted tests of cognition and standardized IQ tests in Meldrum's cohort as these children reach school age. The results could offer some insight into the role of intrauterine exposure; the cord blood DHA level in these children indicated exposure was much higher than in the USA and duration of DHA and ARA supplementation in infancy.

Van der Merwe et al. studied breastfed infants supplemented with either fish oil capsules or olive oil from 3 to 9 months of age. Cognitive development was assessed at 12 months of age using two tests. No differences were observed between the two groups, however an effect cannot be ruled out because the Willatt's test was given when children were quite old and the duration of supplementation was relatively short.

In summary, the study of Colombo et al. suggested that global tests of language and other aspects of development at 18 months do not capture positive effects of DHA and ARA supplementation even though higher performance on more targeted tests was found in infancy and later in childhood. The two studies that provided fish oil as capsules to infants found more DHA in circulating lipids (plasma or erythrocyte), but the large dose of fish oil provided did not prevent a decline in DHA from that found in cord erythrocytes in one study. Not only was the duration of supplementation shorter, but the amount of DHA absorbed may have been much less than from infant formula in the study by Colombo et al.

Micronutrient Studies: Methyl Donors

Choline intake during pregnancy and child cognition at age 7 years

Boeke CE[1,2], Gillman MW[3], Hughes MD[4], Rifas-Shiman SL[3], Villamor E[1,5], Oken E[3]

[1]Departments of Nutrition and Epidemiology, Harvard School of Public Health, Boston, MA, USA; [2]Channing Division of Network Medicine, Brigham and Women's Hospital, Boston, MA, USA; [3]Obesity Prevention Program, Department of Population Medicine, Harvard Medical School and Hard Pilgrim Health Care Institute, Boston, MA, USA; [4]Department of Biostatistics, Harvard School of Public Health, Boston, MA, USA; [5]Department of Epidemiology, School of Public Health, University of Michigan, Ann Arbor, MI, USA

Am J Epidemiol 2013; 177: 1338–1347

Background: Choline, B_{12}, folate and betaine are methyl donors that are proposed to be important for early development and function of the central nervous system. For example, animal models have shown that choline is important for cholinergic transmission and that choline improves offspring memory. The purpose of this study was to assess the relationship between methyl donors in maternal diet during the second trimester and cognition in the offspring at 7 years of age.

Methods: The sample was drawn from participants in the prospective observational longitudinal Project Viva cohort designed to examine the impact of prenatal exposures on offspring growth and development. Enrollment occurred at the first obstetric office visit. At the first- and second-trimester study visits, a food frequency questionnaire was used to collect maternal dietary data. At age 7 years, offspring completed the Wide Range Assessment of Memory and Learning Second Edition (WRAML2), the Design and Picture Memory subtests (assesses visuospatial memory) and the Kaufman Brief Intelligence Test, Second Edition (KBIT-2) to assess verbal and non-verbal IQ. Mothers completed the KBIT-2 as well, and the maternal KBIT-2 score was used as a covariate in the analyses.

Results: A total of 895 mother-child pairs completed this study. After controlling for confounding variables, maternal choline intake during the second trimester was related to offspring WRAML2 scores. Children exposed in utero to the highest quartile of choline intake when compared to the lowest quartile of intake, had scores that were 1.4 points greater. Associations with cognitive test scores were found in separate bivariate models for B_{12}, betaine and folate, however, the effect disappeared when all were included in one model. Other associations approached significance including a positive relationship between first-trimester maternal choline intake and WRAML2 (p = 0.08) and second-trimester maternal choline intake and the child's non-verbal KBIT-2 score (p = 0.06).

Conclusion: Second-trimester maternal choline intake was related to improved offspring memory score at age 7 years. No other nutrients were related to offspring cognition. Measurement of these methyl donors in maternal serum would be of interest to determine if these can be used as biomarkers for intake.

Phosphatidylcholine supplementation in pregnant women consuming moderate choline diets does not enhance infant cognitive function: a randomized, double-blind, placebo-controlled trial

Cheatham CL[1,4], Goldman BD[1,2], Fischer LM[3], da Costa KA[3], Reznick JS[1,2], Zeisel SH[3,4]

[1]Department of Psychology, University of North Carolina at Chapel Hill, Chapel Hill, NC, USA; [2]FPG Child Development Institute, University of North Carolina at Chapel Hill, Chapel Hill, NC, USA; [3]Department of Nutrition, School of Public Health and School of Medicine, University of North Carolina at Chapel Hill, Chapel Hill, NC, USA; [4]Nutrition Research Institute, University of North Carolina at Chapel Hill, Kannapolis, NC, USA

Am J Clin Nutr 2012; 96: 1465–1472

Background: Choline is an essential nutrient important for fetal neurocognitive development. Safety of choline supplementation and optimal levels needed to ensure appropriate fetal neurocognitive development is unknown. The purpose was to assess the safety and efficacy of choline supplementation during pregnancy and breastfeeding and determine the relationship between choline supplementation and early infant cognitive development.

Methods: 140 pregnant women participated in this randomized, double-blind controlled trial. Participants were randomized to the intervention (CHL; 750 mg choline/day) or to the control group (CON; consumed equivalent amounts of corn oil). Women who consented for the study were asked to consume the gel caps from 18 weeks of gestation to 90 days postpartum and planned to breastfeed for ≥90 days. Maternal choline intake was estimated from 3-day food records obtained at 30 weeks of gestation and 45 days postpartum. Infant cognitive testing occurred at 10 and 12 months. Short-term visuospatial memory, long-term episodic memory using an imitation paradigm, language development (MacArthur-Bates Short Form Vocabulary Checklist Level I) and global development (The Mullen Scales of Early Learning) were assessed.

Results: No differences between groups were found for cognitive tests. All infants were breastfed for a minimum of 45 days. No differences between groups were found for adverse events related to choline supplementation. Maternal dietary intake of choline at 30 weeks of gestation and 45 days postpartum did not differ between groups and represented ~80% of recommended intake during pregnancy and 65% of recommended intake during breastfeeding.

Conclusion: Supplementation above and beyond recommendation did not provide offspring neurocognitive developmental advantages at 10 and 12 months. There were no adverse events related to choline supplementation in this population. Future studies should assess maternal serum values for nutrients and have a longer follow-up period for offspring cognitive assessment.

Serum folate but not vitamin B_{12} concentrations are positively associated with cognitive test scores in children aged 6–16 years

Nguyen CT, Gracely EJ, Lee BK

Drexel University, School of Public Health, Philadelphia, PA, USA

J Nutr 2013; 143: 500–504

Background: There is limited evidence suggesting that folate and B_{12} are important for infant cognitive development. Few studies have explored if micronutrient status is related to cognitive performance in childhood. The purpose was to examine the relationship between folate and B_{12} status and cognitive function in 6- to 16-year-olds.

Methods: These data were part of the NHANES III (1988–1994) cohort studied prior to widespread fortification of folate in food. This survey is a representative cross-sectional randomly sampled population from the United States. A total of 5,365 children had blood folate and B_{12} analysis. The Wechsler Intelligence Scale for Children-Revised (WISC-R) and the Wide Range Achievement Test-Revised (WRAT-R) were administered by trained personnel to test cognitive function.

Results: A positive association was found between folate status and reading and block design scores after adjusting for potential confounders. When compared to the reference population, those with folate levels in the fourth quartile had reading scores that were 3.28 points higher and block design scores that were 0.64 points higher. No association was found between B_{12} and any of the cognitive tests.

Conclusion: This was the first study to assess serum micronutrient levels in relation to cognition in children. Higher folate but not vitamin B_{12} status related to higher cognitive performance.

Cobalamin and folate status predicts mental development scores in North Indian children 12–18 months of age

Strand TA[1,3,4], Taneja S[5,6], Ueland PM[2,7], Refsum H[8], Bahl R[9], Schneede J[10], Sommerfelt H[1,4], Bhandari N[5,6]

[1]Centre for International Health, University of Bergen, Bergen, Norway; [2]Institute of Medicine, University of Bergen, Bergen, Norway; [3]Medical Microbiology, Innlandet Hospital Trust, Lillehammer, Norway; [4]Division of Infectious Disease Control, Norwegian Institute of Public Health, Oslo, Norway; [5]All India Institute of Medical Sciences, New Delhi, India; [6]Society for Applied Studies, New Delhi, India; [7]Haukeland University Hospital, Bergen, Norway; [8]Department of Nutrition, Institute of Basic Medical Sciences, University of Oslo, Oslo, Norway and Department of Pharmacology, University of Oxford, Oxford, UK; [9]Department of Child and Adolescent Health and Development, WHO, Geneva, Switzerland; [10]Department of Clinical Pharmacology, University of Umea, Umea, Sweden

Am J Clin Nutr 2013; 97: 310–317

Background: Micronutrient deficiencies can impair infant neurocognitive development. This is more common in poor countries with limited access to proper infant nutrition or where maternal vegan diets are common. The purpose was to examine the relationship between infant serum status for folate, B_{12}, total homocysteine and methylmalonic acid and cognitive scores in North Indian infants.

Methods: These outcomes were secondary aims of a parent trial to assess the effectiveness of zinc supplementation on illness rate. 571 children were assessed between 12 and 18 months of age and again 4 months later. Blood was collected at the first visit and subsets of the Bayley developmental index (Mental Development Index (MDI) and Psychomotor Development Index (PDI)) were administered at both visits to assess cognitive development.

Results: Zinc supplementation had no effect on cognition in the primary study. Higher serum homocysteine and methylmalonic acid concentrations predicted lower MDI at follow-up: For every twofold increase in the concentrations of homocysteine and methylmalonic acid, the MDI scored decreased by 2.0 (95% CI 0.5–3.4; $p = 0.007$) and 1.1 (95% CI 0.3–1.8; $p = 0.004$), respectively. Folate predicted MDI at baseline and follow-up ($\beta = 1.3$, $p = 0.02$ and $\beta = 1.6$, $p = 0.003$, respectively) only in those infants with a serum B_{12} status >25th percentile.

Conclusion: Higher levels of homocysteine and methylmalonic acid are related to poorer infant neurocognitive development. Folate was related to better cognitive scores only in those infants with a higher B_{12} status. Trials are needed to test the effectiveness of B_{12} and folate supplementation on cognitive development in children at risk for deficiency. A risk factor for B_{12} deficiency may have been continued breastfeeding. 74% were still breastfed at a mean of 14.9 months.

Maternal intake of methyl-donor nutrient and child cognition at 3 years of age

Villamor E[1,2], Rifas-Shiman SL[3], Gillman MW[2,3], Oken E[3]

[1]Department of Epidemiology, School of Public Health, University of Michigan, Ann Arbor, MI, USA; [2]Department of Nutrition, Harvard School of Public Health, Boston, MA, USA; [3]Obesity Prevention Program, Department of Population Medicine, Harvard Medical School and Hard Pilgrim Health Care Institute, Boston, MA, USA

Paediatr Perinat Epidemiol 2012; 26: 328–335

Background: Methylation reactions are important for development and function of the nervous system. Nutrients that act as methyl donors (B_{12}, folate, choline and betaine) have been suggested to be important for neurocognitive development. The purpose of this study was to assess the maternal dietary intake of methyl-donor nutrients during pregnancy and compare them to values to offspring cognitive development at age 3 years.

Methods: Women were participants in the prospective observational longitudinal Project Viva cohort designed to examine the impact of prenatal exposures on offspring growth and development. Women were enrolled early in pregnancy and food frequency questionnaires were used to collect maternal dietary data throughout pregnancy. At 3 years of age, offspring completed the Peabody Picture Vocabulary Test III (PPVT-III) and the Wide Range Assessment of Visual Motor abilities (WRAVMA).

Results: A total of 1,210 participants were included in this analysis. When controlling for confounding variables, maternal folate intake from food and supplements during the first trimester was related to offspring PPVT-III scores. A 600 µg/day increase in maternal folate intake was associated with an increase of 1.6 points on the PPVT-III. A small negative association was observed between maternal second-trimester vitamin B_{12} intake and the PPVT-III. For every increase of maternal B_{12} intake by 2.6 µg/day, a 0.4-point score decrease was predicted for the PPVT-III. No relationship was found between any methyl-donor nutrient and the score on the WRAVMA.

Conclusion: Maternal dietary folate intake was related to improved neurocognitive scores in off-spring in early childhood. Future studies assessing serum levels of maternal methyl-donor nutrients are needed to confirm these findings.

Comments Five papers published this past year studied status of methyl donors (choline, betaine, folate and vitamin B_{12}) and cognition. A cohort of 6- to 16-year-old children from NHANES III (before widespread fortification of food with folate) was evaluated for a relationship between serum folate or vitamin B_{12} and cognition. Serum folate but not vitamin B_{12} concentration was related to higher cognitive performance. Similarly, higher serum folate was related to higher BSID MDI scores in a study of North Indian infants and toddlers in those with a vitamin B_{12} concentration above the 25th percentile. However, higher homocysteine and methylmalonic acid (both associated with low methyl donor status) were associated with lower BSID MDI scores.

Villamor et al. estimated methyl donor intake in pregnant Bostonian women from food and supplements in the Project VIVA cohort (1,210 participants) and child cognitive performance at 3 years of age. Scores on the PPVT-III were higher with higher maternal folate intake in the first trimester of pregnancy, however maternal vitamin B_{12} intake was associated with a small decrease in the PPVT-III. Boeke et al. estimated maternal intake of methyl donors in the second trimester and compared this to off-spring cognition at 7 years measured by the WRAML2 and other cognitive tests. Choline intake, but not intake of other methyl donors, correlated with higher memory at 7 years. Cheatham et al. supplemented pregnant women with choline (750 mg/day) during the last half of pregnancy and the first 3 months of lactation but did not find any neurocognitive development advantage at 10 and 12 months although women in the study consumed good amounts of dietary choline.

Several of these studies support the idea that low maternal methyl donor intake, particularly folate and choline, during intrauterine development result in lower developmental scores, however future studies should control for socioeconomic status as intake of folate and vitamin B_{12} and possibly other methyl donors is linked to income and education.

Micronutrient Studies: Iron, Vitamin A and Iodine

Iron-deficiency anemia in infancy and poorer cognitive inhibitory control at age 10 years

Algarin C[1], Nelson CA[2], Peirano P[1], Westerlund A[2], Reyes S[1], Lozoff B[3]

[1]Sleep and Functional Neurobiology Laboratory, Institute of Nutrition and Food Technology, University of Chile, Santiago, Chile; [2]Developmental Medicine Research, Harvard Medical School, Children's Hospital Boston, DMC Laboratories of Cognitive Neuroscience, Boston, MA, USA; [3]Center for Human Growth and Development, University of Michigan, Ann Arbor, MI, USA

Dev Med Child Neurol 2013; 55: 453–458

Background: Iron is an important micronutrient for brain development, specifically the regions of the brain related to inhibitory control and response inhibition. It is unknown if exposure to iron-deficiency anemia (IDA) during infancy impairs these functions long term. The purpose of the study was to compare cognitive performance of 10-year-olds diagnosed with compared to without IDA during infancy on tasks that assess executive function.

Methods: This was a follow-up to a study assessing the behavioral, developmental and neurofunctional effects of IDA during infancy in a Chilean population. Anemia was defined as hemoglobin <100 g/l at 6 months or <110 g/l at 12 or 18 months of age. IDA was treated with 15 or 30 mg/day of iron depending on age. Children with IDA at age 10 were excluded from the study. A go/no-go task assessed inhibition and event-related potentials (ERPs), electro-oculography and electroencephalography were recorded.

Results: When compared to children without IDA during infancy, children diagnosed with IDA during infancy had slower reaction times, decreased accuracy, longer latency to the N2 peak and a smaller P300 amplitude.

Conclusion: Children exposed to IDA during infancy showed poorer scores on neurocognitive tests. These findings suggest that even when anemia is corrected early, IDA leads to cognitive deficits in childhood.

Cognitive and motor skills in school-aged children following maternal vitamin A supplementation during pregnancy in rural Nepal: a follow-up of a placebo-controlled, randomized cohort

Buckley GJ[1], Murray-Kolb LE[2], Khatry SK[3], LeClerq SC[1], Wu L, West KP[1], Christian P[1]

[1]Center for Human Nutrition, Johns Hopkins Bloomberg School of Public Health, Baltimore, MA, USA; [2]Department of Nutritional Sciences, The Pennsylvania State University, University Park, PA, USA; [3]Nepal Nutrition Intervention Project, Sarlahi, Nepal Netra Jyoti Sangh, Tripureswor, Kathmandu, Nepal

BMJ Open 2013; 3: e002000

Background: Retinoic acid is vital for fetal neural development, in particular for neural tube formation, neuron development and synaptic signaling. Vitamin A deficiency is common in poor pregnant women from underdeveloped countries. The purpose is to examine the long-term impact of perinatal vitamin A supplementation on offspring cognitive and motor development at 10–13 years of age.

Methods: The original study was a cluster randomized, placebo-controlled trial. Married women of reproductive age were randomized by village to treatment (TRT) or control (CON). The TRT group received weekly oral doses of vitamin A (7,000 μg retinol equivalents) during a continuous period of 3.5 years. Cognition was assessed using the Universal Nonverbal Intelligence Test (UNIT) and Movement Assessment Battery for Children (MABC) assessed motor ability.

Results: 390 children completed follow-up. No group differences were found for UNIT (mean difference –1.07; p = 0.78) or MABC scores (mean difference 0.18; p = 0.15), however a greater proportion of children in the CON had repeated a grade when compared to the TRT group (28 vs. 16.7%; p = 0.01), suggesting some functional impairment.

Conclusion: At 10 to 13 years of age, no effect of vitamin A supplementation during pregnancy on cognitive or motor development was found. Periconceptual vitamin A supplementation was not effective at improving neurocognitive or motor skills in offspring in childhood.

Effect of inadequate iodine status in UK pregnant women on cognitive outcomes in their children: results from the Avon Longitudinal Study of Parents and Children (ALSPAC)

Bath SC[1], Steer CD[2], Golding J[2], Emmett P[2], Rayman MP[1]

[1]Department of Nutritional Sciences, Faculty of Health and Medical Sciences, University of Surry, Guildford, UK; [2]Centre for Child and Adolescent Health, School of Social and Community Medicine, University of Bristol, Bristol, UK

Lancet 2013; 382: 331–337

Background: Iodine is crucial for fetal neurocognitive development. Iodine deficiency may be present in otherwise well-nourished populations. The purpose was to examine the relationship between maternal iodine status during early pregnancy and offspring neurocognitive development in the UK. *Method:* Data were drawn from the Avon Longitudinal Study of Parents and Children. A total of 1,040 mother-child pairs were used for this analysis. Urinary iodine concentration was measured late in the first trimester (median 10 weeks) and creatinine was used to correct for urine volume (iodine:creatinine ratio). The maternal iodine:creatinine ratio was dichotomized to values <150 μg/g (deficient) or ≥150 μg/g (sufficient). The Wechsler Intelligence Scale for Children was used to assess offspring IQ at 8 years of age. One year later, the Neale Analysis of Reading Ability was administered to test reading speed, accuracy and comprehension.
Results: A greater proportion of children born to mothers with iodine deficiency in the first trimester of pregnancy had suboptimal cognitive performance compared to children born to mothers who were iodine-sufficient. After adjusting for all known confounding variables, offspring exposed to iodine deficiency were 1.4–1.69 times more likely to have scores in the lowest quartile for verbal IQ, reading accuracy and reading comprehension (p < 0.03). When the deficient iodine category was subdivided further (<50 or 50–150 μg/g), cognitive scores were worse with decreasing maternal iodine status.
Conclusion: Poor maternal iodine status early in pregnancy is associated with impaired cognitive development in offspring during childhood. Further studies controlling maternal intake of iodine during pregnancy are needed to verify these findings.

Mild iodine deficiency during pregnancy is associated with reduced educational outcomes in the offspring: 9-year follow-up of the gestational iodine cohort

Hynes KL[1], Oahal P[1], Hay I[2], Burgess JR[3,4]

[1]Menzies Research Institute Tasmania, University of Tasmania, Sandy Bay, TAS, Australia; [2]Faculty of Education, University of Tasmania, Sandy Bay, TAS, Australia; [3]School of Medicine, University of Tasmania, Sandy Bay, TAS, Australia; [4]Department of Endocrinology, Royal Hobart Hospital, Hobart, TAS, Australia

J Clin Endocrinol Metab 2013; 98: 1954–1962

Background: Iodine is an important micronutrient for normal fetal and childhood neurocognitive development. The few studies that have examined maternal iodine deficiency during pregnancy in relation to offspring cognitive development have found mixed results. The purpose of this study was to examine the impact of maternal iodine deficiency on educational outcomes of the offspring at 9 years of age.

Methods: This was a follow-up study assessing the impact of iodine deficiency during pregnancy. Maternal iodine deficiency was defined as a urinary iodine concentration <150 µg/l diagnosed anytime during pregnancy and treated. Educational outcomes were measured and included Australian and Tasmanian standardized educational tests that assess spelling, grammar, English literacy, reading, writing and mathematics/numeracy.

Results: Follow-up data was available for 228 children. In unadjusted analysis, offspring of mothers with iodine deficiency had lower spelling, grammar and English literacy scores compared to offspring of women who were iodine-sufficient. However, after adjusting for biological and socioeconomic factors, only spelling scores remained significant. Offspring of iodine-deficient mothers had a 38.6-point reduction (95% CI –65.6 to –11.6; p = 0.005) in spelling scores when compared to offspring not exposed to iodine deficiency.

Conclusion: These results suggest expose to gestational iodine deficiency has long-term cognitive effects even when iodine insufficiency is corrected during childhood.

Comments   Only one report of iron-deficiency anemia (IDA) and cognition was published this year. Algarin et al. studied a group of 10-year-old Chileans diagnosed with IDA and treated during infancy and compared them to a group without IDA. Even though treated for IDA in infancy, IDA during infancy was linked to cognitive and electrophysiological impairment at 10 years of age.

The effects of perinatal vitamin A supplementation on cognitive development in 10- to 13-year-old children were evaluated in a cohort from rural Nepal. No differences were found on non-verbal IQ and motor ability using standardized tests between children in the villages randomized to provide vitamin A to women of reproductive age and villages not randomized to vitamin A. The only difference found was that fewer children had to repeat a grade in school if they were born in a village given treatment. Given the importance of good vitamin A status for immune function, it would have been helpful to have information on missed school days to determine if this finding was related to a cognitive effect or that the children were simply healthier and better able to attend school.

The role of iodine status during pregnancy was evaluated in two studies this year – one conducted in the UK ALSPAC cohort and one conducted in Australia and Tasmania. Both found adverse effects on cognitive function of offspring of women with iodine deficiency during pregnancy (characterized as a urinary iodine of <150 g/µg of creatinine or <150 µg/l for these respective studies). IQ was determined with the WISC in the ALSPAC cohort when children were 8 years of age; a test of writing ability was conducted at 9 years of age. Verbal IQ, reading accuracy and reading comprehension were more likely to be in the lowest quartile for offspring of iodine-deficient mothers. The Australian and Tasmanian cohort were tested on standardized education tests with only spelling scores significantly lower in offspring of iodine-deficient compared to iodine-sufficient women at 9 years of age.

Overall Summary: The majority of the studies published this year used well-established cognitive assessments or assessments targeted to specific behavioral domains and were done at ages when the assessments could be used to discriminate between children's performance (tests were age-appropriate, but not too easy or too difficult). Many also used multiple measures of cognitive function and tested children at school age when cognition is better measured. It is also heartening that most controlled for potentially influential variables to minimize the chances that findings were due to other forms of deprivation. The studies for the most part studied large cohorts and appear to be adequately powered to accept or reject the null hypothesis. These are all signs of increasing sophistication in studies of nutrition and cognitive development compared to the past, and they suggest productive collaboration between nutrition and developmental scientists. The overall impression left by studies published this year is that many nutrient deficiencies early in development can lead to adverse effects on cognitive development at school age. However, it is clear that some of these studies have only opened the door. More studies are needed to provide the quality of evidence needed to create public policy.

Koletzko B, Shamir R, Turck D, Phillip M (eds): Nutrition and Growth: Yearbook 2014.
World Rev Nutr Diet. Basel, Karger, 2014, vol 109, pp 54–88 (DOI: 10.1159/000356108)

Nutrition and Growth in Chronic Diseases

Corina Hartman[1,2], Mabrouka A. Altowati[3], S. Faisal Ahmed[3] and
Raanan Shamir[1,2]

[1] Institute of Gastroenterology, Nutrition and Liver Diseases, Schneider Children's Medical Center of Israel,
Clalit Health Services, Petach-Tikva, Israel
[2] Sackler School of Medicine, Tel Aviv University, Tel Aviv, Israel
[3] Developmental Endocrinology Research Group, Royal Hospital for Sick Children, Glasgow, UK

Both acute and chronic diseases can affect nutritional status and growth. Acute disease exerts reversible effects on rate of weight gain whereas chronic disease may result in changes in weight and height gain with potential long-lasting effects including poor response to disease treatment and reduced final adult height. Nutritional support is needed in many different clinical conditions ranging from children with anorexia associated with acute infectious disease to malnourished children with chronic disease. Administration of appropriate nutritional support is conditioned by the understanding of the multiple changes that take place in dietary intake, metabolic rate and changes in physical activity. Proper nutritional support should both prevent weight loss in the short term and promote appropriate growth in the long term. Chronic disease may also affect pubertal progress which in turn may have led to a number of effects including poor growth. This chapter presents a selection of last year's publications that focused on the nutritional support and growth in several of the most common chronic diseases of children.

Innate dysfunction promotes linear growth failure in pediatric Crohn's disease and growth hormone resistance in murine ileitis

D'Mello S[1], Trauernicht A[1], Ryan A[1], Bonkowski E[1], Willson T[1,3], Trapnell BC[2], Frank SJ[4], Kugasathan S[5], Denson LA[1,3]

[1]Gastroenterology, Hepatology, and Nutrition, Cincinnati Children's Hospital Medical Center and the University of Cincinnati College of Medicine, University of Cincinnati, Cincinnati, OH, USA; [2]Pulmonary Biology, Cincinnati Children's Hospital Medical Center and the University of Cincinnati College of Medicine, University of Cincinnati, Cincinnati, OH, USA; [3]Department of Cancer and Cell Biology, University of Cincinnati, Cincinnati, OH, USA; [4]Department of Medicine, University of Alabama at Birmingham School of Medicine, and Medical Service, Birmingham VA Medical Center, Birmingham, AL, USA; [5]Department of Pediatrics, Emory University School of Medicine, Atlanta, GA, USA

Inflamm Bowel Dis 2012; 18: 236–245

Background: A previous study by the same authors suggested that patients with elevated granulocyte macrophage colony-stimulating factor autoantibodies (GM-CSF Ab) are more likely to experience complicated ileal disease requiring surgery. The aim of this report was to investigate any association between GM-CSF Ab and CARD15 risk allele (C15+GMAb+) with growth failure in CD, and growth hormone (GH) resistance in a model of murine ileitis.

Methods: 229 children with Crohn's disease (CD) recruited at two sites had CARD15 genotype, serum GM-CSF Ab, GH-binding protein (GHBP), height (HtSDS) and weight (WtSDS) z-scores evaluated at diagnosis. There were 45 patients with both a CARD15 risk allele and elevated GM-CSF Ab (C15+GMAb+) and 184 patients with one or neither, and served as controls. Age at diagnosis, age at blood sample collection, gender, and frequency of moderate-to-severe disease activity at diagnosis were similar between the groups. Ileitis was induced in CARD15-deficient mice by GM-CSF neutralization and NSAID exposure. Hepatic GH receptor (GHr) abundance and GH-dependent Stat5 activation were determined by Western blot and IGF-1 mRNA expression by real-time PCR.

Results: Patients with both elevated GM-CSF Ab/CARD15 have reduced mean HtSDS (–0.48) at diagnosis compared to –0.07 in the disease control cohort (p < 0.05). The proportion of growth retardation (HtSDS ≤–1) and growth failure (HtSDS ≤–1.8) were higher in the C15+GMAb+ group (38 and 16%, respectively) when compared to controls (18 and 6%). No difference was found in WtSDS between groups. Circulating GHBP, as a surrogate indicator for tissue GHR abundance, was significantly decreased in the C15+GMAb+ group. In univariate analysis, the C15+GMAb+ state was strongly associated with small bowel location. The C15+GMAb+ state was not associated with WtSDS. In stepwise multivariate analysis, the inclusion of small bowel location reduced the effect of C15+GMAb+ state upon HtSDS, while the inclusion of WtSDS reduced the effect of small bowel location upon HtSDS. Hepatic GHR abundance and GH induction of Stat5 tyrosine phosphorylation and IGF-1 mRNA expression in male CARD15-deficient mice with ileitis was reduced.

Conclusion: The study showed that defects in innate immunity that are due to the presence of GM-CSF Ab in the CARD15-deficient host are associated with growth impairment in CD and hepatic GH resistance in murine ileitis. Growth failure in patients with CD and GH resistance in the animal model occurred in the absence of differences in inflammation or weight, suggesting a specific effect of the C15+GMAb+ state.

Comments Several reports have investigated the possible mechanisms implicated in growth impairment in children with CD. However, many gaps still exist in our knowledge of this important complication. Studies have consistently shown that proximal small bowel disease location is associated with reduced linear growth [1, 2]. Male gender has also been associated with a predisposition to reduce linear growth [1, 2]. In this study, growth impairment in patients and GH resistance in the animal model occurred in the absence of differences in inflammatory cytokines (TNF-α and IL-6) or weight between two groups. Defective barrier function in small intestine has been suggested to directly induce GH resistance and growth failure. The authors highlight that in IBD, patient-dependent factors may also modulate growth independent of inflammation. This link between the gastrointestinal system and growth may also exist in conditions other than IBD.

Serum antibodies and anthropometric data at diagnosis in pediatric Crohn's disease

Trauernicht AK, Steiner SJ

Division of Pediatric Gastroenterology/Hepatology/Nutrition, James Whitcomb Riley Hospital for Children, Indiana University School of Medicine, Indianapolis, IN, USA

Dig Dis Sci 2012; 57: 1020–1025

Background: Patients diagnosed with IBD have variable immune responses to microbial antigens including the formation of antibodies to *Escherichia coli* outer-membrane protein C (OmpC) and *Saccharomyces cerevisiae* (ASCA), and autoantigens to perinuclear antineutrophil antibody (pANCA)/neutrophil-specific nuclear autoantibodies (NSNA). These serum immune responses may correlate with the location of the disease and may be used to predict disease progression. An increased number of serum immune responses and an increased level of response are positively correlated with the severity of the disease. In this research the authors evaluated serum immune responses and anthropometric measurement at the time of initial diagnosis for pediatric CD patients.
Methods: This retrospective report looked at height and weight z-score in 102 children (mean age 11.9 years) with CD before diagnosis and compared the anthropometric data among groups according to presence of specific antibodies at time of diagnosis.
Results: The authors showed that the mean weight and height z-score were lower in subjects with positive ASCA titers than in patients without any antibodies present.
Conclusion: The newly diagnosed CD patients with positive ASCA antibodies had lower mean height and weight z-scores. The authors claimed that some groups of children with CD can be at greater risk of growth impairment before diagnosis.

Comments This is the first report which examines the correlation between growth data at the time of diagnosis and serum immune responses in children with IBD. Although it is possible that this information may allow improvement in tailoring of therapy to optimize growth outcome in an individualized manner, there is a need to perform some longitudinal studies to confirm this impression. These data also highlight the need to a better understanding of the interaction between circulating markers of inflammation and the endocrine and paracrine control of growth.

Mathematical modeling to restore circulating IGF-1 concentrations in children with Crohn's disease-induced growth failure: a pharmacokinetic study

Rao A[1], Standing JF[2], Naik S[1], Savage MO[3], Sanderson IR[1]

[1]Centre for Digestive Diseases, Blizard Institute, Barts and The London School of Medicine and Dentistry, Queen Mary, University of London, London, UK; [2]Infectious Diseases and Microbiology Unit, Institute of Child Health, University College London, London, UK; [3]Centre for Endocrinology, William Harvey Research Institute, Barts and The London School of Medicine and Dentistry, Queen Mary, University of London, London, UK

BMJ 2013; 3: 1–11

Background: Around a third of the children with CD experience impairment in linear growth, caused in part by undernutrition and in part by the direct effects of inflammation on growth. Children with active CD have high cytokine levels and low IGF-1. In vitro studies have shown a strong link between inflammatory cytokines, IGF-1 and poor growth and reported of a state of functional GH insensitivity secondary to decreased response of IGF-1 to GH. Control of inflammation/ significant reduction in cytokine levels and subsequent increase in IGF-1 hence are the first steps in improving growth. However, in some of children, inflammation remains intractable despite use of advanced therapy and there is no agreed growth-promoting treatment for them. Recently, recombinant human IGF-1 (rhIGF-1) has been used as a growth-promoting therapy for children with GH insensitivity syndrome. This group of researchers hypothesized that IGF-1 concentration in children with active CD and poor linear growth could be restored by administration of rhIGF-1. The difficulty is that restoring the IGF-1 level within a normal range is not straightforward and high and sustained IGF-1 levels over time have been associated with an increased incidence of colon cancer in adults with acromegaly. This could, in theory, represent an additional hazard for children with CD, already exposed to chronic inflammation, also a risk factor for intestinal cancer. The authors postulate that developing a mathematical model for IGF-1 treatment may better define the dosing regimen which restores IGF-1 concentration to a normal range without the further risk of cancer.

Methods: This was a pharmacokinetics intervention study in 8 children over 10 years with active CD (C-reactive protein >10 mg/l or erythrocyte sedimentation rate >25 mm/h) and height velocity SDS <−2 SDS. Subcutaneous rhIGF-1 (120 µg/kg) per dose was given over two admissions: the first as a single dose and the second over 5 days as twice-daily doses. The primary endpoint was a significant increase in serum IGF-1.

Results: Twice-daily subcutaneous rhIGF-1 led to a significant increase of circulating IGF-1 over a sustained period with low variability between peaks. In covariate analysis, disease activity significantly reduces endogenous production of IGF-1.

Conclusion: IGF-1 dosing using a mathematical model including age, weight and disease activity, normalized the IGF-1 level in over 95% of children with CD and achieved levels below +2.5 SDS of normal population mean, a level not associated with cancer risk.

Comments The study is the first interventional study on IGF-1 treatment in children with CD. The authors used a mathematical model to determine the dose of rhIGF-1 that maintained serum IGF-1 level within the physiological range. The dosing schedule which reflects the age dependency of circulating IGF-1 in normal children and the state of GH resistance in children with CD was 21 + 1 µg/kg/PCDAI point for the 10- to 12-year-olds and 41 + 1.4 µg/kg/PCDAI point for the 12- to 14-year-olds. Growth-promoting therapies such as rhGH, rhIGF-1 or the two in combination are currently being explored as possible methods of promoting growth in children with disease-related growth retardation and this study may assist in the design of future clinical trials. The study also showed that the extent of protein-losing enteropathy measured by fecal α_1-antitrypsin level did not alter IGF-1 or IGFBP-3 levels. Administration of rhIGF-1 to children with a decreased level of IGFBP-3 may lead to increased free IGF-1 but this was not evaluated in this study. However, the authors stated that the level of IGFBP-3 was not severely depressed as it remained with 2 SDs of normal even in the most severely affected cases.

Nutrition and Growth

Clinical progress in the two years following a course of exclusive enteral nutrition in 109 paediatric patients with Crohn's disease

Cameron FL[1], Gerasimidis K[2], Papangelou A[2], Missiou D[2], Garrick V[1], Cardigan T[1], Buchanan E[1], Barclay AR[1], McGrogan P[1], Russell RK[1]

[1]Department of Paediatric Gastroenterology, Hepatology and Nutrition, Royal Hospital for Sick Children, Glasgow, UK; [2]Life Course Nutrition and Health, Centre for Population and Health Sciences, Institute of Health and Wellbeing, College of Medicine, Veterinary and Life Sciences, University of Glasgow, Glasgow, UK

Aliment Pharmacol Ther 2013; 37: 622–629

Background: Exclusive enteral nutrition (EEN) is increasingly considered an effective initial method of controlling inflammation in children with active CD. This paper investigates the short- and long-term outcome of EEN on both the clinical course of disease and growth indices.
Methods: In this study, case notes of 109 (68 males) newly diagnosed CD patients with a median age 11.2 years who completed an 8-week course of EEN were retrospectively reviewed. Data on demographics, growth, disease characteristics and inflammatory markers (albumin, CRP, ESR and platelets) were collected at EEN initiation and at 1, 2, 6, 12 and 24 months after initiation of therapy.
Results: In total, 65 patients were in remission, 32 improved, and 12 had no improvement after 8 weeks of EEN. By 4 weeks, weight SDS, BMI SDS and all inflammatory markers improved. Relapses occurred in 63/109 (58%) during follow-up and 44/63 (70%) responded to a second course of EEN. Although use of EEN increased height velocity up to 6 months in responders, it was not associated with improvement in HtSDS over 24 months. Use of azathioprine within 6 months of diagnosis also did not show any benefit in terms of improvement height outcomes at 24 months.
Conclusion: An 8-week course of EEN resulted in an improvement in weight parameters up to 2 years but not in height z-score.

Comments This relatively large retrospective study confirms previous observations that despite disease remission (as assessed by global patient assessment in combination with clinical parameters), improvement in weight and short-term improvement in height velocity, the use of EEN may not be associated with a sustained improvement in HtSDS over the longer term. Thus, there is a need to continue investigating novel forms of growth promotion in these children. The authors also point out that improvement in weight and inflammatory markers was already present by 4 weeks, thus questioning the need for 8 weeks of EEN.

Biologics and Growth

Partial normalization of pubertal timing in female mice with DSS colitis treated with anti-TNF-α antibody

DeBoer MD, Steinman J, Li Y

Division of Pediatric Endocrinology, University of Virginia, Charlottesville, VA, USA

J Gastroenterol 2012; 47: 647–654

Background: Delayed puberty is a common concern for children with IBD, and especially CD, and is associated with inadequate growth, defective bone mineralization and poor self-esteem. Currently, biologic agents are the mainstay in children with more severe forms of IBD resistant to conventional treatment. Biologic agents are engineered proteins which selectively neutralize or block the effects of different cytokines. One of the commonly used agents is infliximab, a monoclonal antibody to tumor necrosis factor-α (TNF-α). Some studies have reported that the use of infliximab is associated with improved growth in children with CD whose disease improves. However, whether infliximab treatment affects the timing of puberty is not yet clear. This experimental study was designed to determine whether TNF-α antibodies normalize pubertal progress and whether infliximab causes any change in the function of the hypothalamic-pituitary-gonad (HPG) axis in female mice with induced colitis.

Methods: Dextran sodium sulfate (DSS) colitis was induced in 23-day-old female mice and the treatment groups were divided into three groups: control + TNF-α antibodies, DSS-induced colitis + control antibodies, and DSS-induced colitis + TNF-α antibodies. All groups were monitored for the timing of vaginal opening until day 33 of life, when they were euthanized for serum and colon collection.

Results: Timing of vaginal opening in DSS + TNF-α and control + TNF-α antibodies was similar and occurred earlier compared with DSS + control antibody group. Also, DSS + TNF-α antibody had a higher LH level after GnRH stimulation and lower systemic interleukin-6 compared to the DSS + control antibody group. No differences were observed in weight gain, growth, or colon histological inflammatory scores between the three groups over the course of the experiment.

Conclusion: The authors demonstrated that treatment with monoclonal antibodies to TNF-α was associated with partial normalization in the timing of pubertal onset in female mice with DSS colitis.

Comments The authors of this study have previously shown that female mice with DSS colitis had a later timing of vaginal opening than food-restricted mice of the same body weight. In the current study they confirmed this finding and showed that this difference persisted in spite of similar weight gain and circulating leptin. The only difference was in the extent of inflammation as assessed by circulating cytokines and gut inflammation. The raised levels of LH in DSS colitis model treated with TNF-α antibodies are intriguing and the authors did not have a good explanation for this. This effect was not observed in the control group suggesting that colitis may sensitize the hypothalamic pituitary axis to GnRH stimulation. The hypothalamic-pituitary-gonadal axis is under negative feedback control by circulating sex steroids and it is possible that the increased responsiveness to GnRH may reflect direct suppression of sex steroid synthesis at the level of the peripheral steroid-secreting organs by the cytokines. The investigators suggest that in humans the use of biologics may be associated with pubertal progress or increased gonadal activity, but this requires further investigation.

Long-term outcome of tumor necrosis factor-α antagonist's treatment in pediatric Crohn's disease

Assa A[1,4], Hartman C[1,4], Weiss B[2,4], Broide E[3,4], Rosenbach Y[1,4], Zevit N[1,4], Bujanover Y[2,4], Shamir R[1,4]

[1]Institute of Gastroenterology, Nutrition and Liver Disease, Schneider Children's Medical Center, Petach-Tikva, Israel; [2]Pediatric Gastroenterology Unit, Edmond and Lily Safra Children's Hospital, Sheba Medical Center, Tel Hashomer, Israel; [3]Pediatric Gastroenterology Unit, Assaf Harofeh Medical Center, Zerifin, Israel; [4]Sackler School of Medicine, Tel Aviv University, Tel Aviv, Israel

J Crohn Colitis 2013; 7: 369–376

Background: The efficacy of infliximab for both induction and maintenance of moderate to severe pediatric CD is widely accredited. However, its effect on optimization of linear growth seems to be variable. Some studies demonstrated a short-term increase in height velocity during infliximab treatment while others showed no significant change during a similar follow-up time. One of the secondary outcomes of this study was to examine the long-term outcome of anti-TNF-α on the growth of children with IBD.

Methods: In this multicenter study, 102 IBD children who received anti-TNF-α therapy at a mean age of 13.4 ± 3.9 years for a median duration of 15 (2–90) months were retrospectively studied. The authors recorded long-term response rates, predictors for loss of response as well as the effect of treatment on anthropometric parameters.

Results: A short-term beneficial response on disease was observed in 91/102 (89%) of the cohort following induction and a prolonged response for more than 6 months occurred in 84/102 (84%). The mean BMI z-score improved significantly in responders (–0.8 to –0.4, p = 0.04) compared to non-responders. A tendency towards enhanced growth velocity was also found in responders compared to non-responders. Only male responders showed a significant increase in height velocity during treatment.

Conclusion: In agreement with the current literature, the study showed that biologic agents were effective and safe in the long term. Furthermore, the clinical response was associated with improved weight and BMI.

Comments   The ability of biologic agents to improve growth and growth failure in children with CD continues to be an area of controversial debate. The growth data from this study needed to be interpreted with caution because of a lack of pubertal growth information. In addition, a large proportion of the cohort patients were on glucocorticoids which may also have affected growth.

The effects of anti-TNF-α treatment with adalimumab on growth in children with Crohn's disease

Malik S[1,2], Ahmed SF[1], Wilson ML[3], Shah N[4], Loganathan S[5], Naik S[6], Bourke B[7], Thomas A[8], Akobeng AK[8], Fagbemi A[8], Wilson DC[3], Russell RK[2]

[1]Bone & Endocrine Research Group, Royal Hospital for Sick Children, Yorkhill, Glasgow, UK; [2]Department of Paediatric Gastroenterology & Nutrition, Royal Hospital for Sick Children, Yorkhill, Glasgow, UK; [3]University of Edinburgh, Child Life and Health, Edinburgh, UK; [4]Great Ormond Street Hospital Paediatric Gastroenterology Department, London, UK; [5]Royal Aberdeen Children's Hospital, Department of Medical Paediatrics, Aberdeen, UK; [6]Bart's and the London Children's Hospital, London, UK; [7]Our Lady's Children's Hospital Crumlin, Children's Research Centre, Dublin, Ireland; [8]Royal Manchester Children's Hospital, Manchester, UK

J Crohn Colitis 2012; 6: 337–344

Background: Adalimumab is a humanized anti-TNF therapy that has been shown to be effective for induction and maintenance of remission for adults with Crohn's disease (CD). Clinical studies of adalimumb in children are relatively limited; no studies have yet examined the effect of adalimumb on growth. In this multicentre retrospective study the authors assessed the influence of adalimumab therapy on growth and disease activity in children with CD.

Methods: Growth and disease activity of 36 children with CD who started adalimumab at a median age of 14.7 years (11.3–16.8) were collected at 6 months before (T–6), at baseline (T0) and 6 months after (T+6) starting adalimumab.

Results: Remission occurred in 28/36 children (78%). 15 children (42%) demonstrated improvement in their growth, median change in height z-score (ΔHtSDS) increased from –0.3 at T0 to +0.3 at T+6. The improvement in ΔHtSDS was more likely in children who achieved remission (ΔHtSDS) increased from –0.2 at T0 to +0.2 at T+6. In those in pubertal Tanner stage II–III, median ΔHtSDS improved from –0.4 at T0 to +0.2 at T+6. In those with immunosuppression background, ΔHtSDS increased from –0.2 at T0 to +0.1 at T+6. When adalimumab was indicated because of infliximab allergy, median ΔHtSDS increased from –0.3 at T0 to +0.3 at T+6. The change in height SDS also improved in children who were on prednisolone when starting adalimumb.

Conclusion: This study showed that the clinical response to adalimumab therapy was associated with an improvement in linear growth in children with CD.

Comments   The results of this study suggest that the use of adalimumab can be helpful in terms of linear growth improvement in children with CD. By looking at the results, growth improvement in this cohort may be credited to both controlling of inflammation and progression of puberty, as the increase in ΔHtSDS was more likely in those who achieved remission as well as in pre-puberty and in-puberty children. However, it is uncertain yet from this study and other studies whether this short-term improvement in linear growth is maintained over a longer period and whether there is an improvement in final height, which is the ultimate objective in any patients with growth impairment. It is anticipated that future efforts will be directed to also explore the effect of biologics on final height in adults with childhood-onset CD.

Growth in children receiving contemporary disease-specific therapy for Crohn's disease

Malik S[1,2], Mason A[1], Bakhshi A[3], Young D[4], Bishop J[2], Garrick V[2], McGrogan P[2], Russell RK[2], Ahmed FS[1]

[1]Department of Child Health, University of Glasgow, Bone and Endocrine Research Group, Royal Hospital for Sick Children, Yorkhill, Glasgow, UK; [2]Department of Paediatric Gastroenterology and Nutrition, University of Glasgow, Royal Hospital for Sick Children, Yorkhill, Glasgow, UK; [3]School of Mathematics and Statistics, University of Glasgow, Glasgow, UK; [4]Department of Statistics and Modelling Science, University of Strathclyde, Glasgow, UK

Arch Dis Child 2012; 97: 698–703

Background: Data from recent studies have shown that despite improvements in therapy, nutrition and a decrease in the use of glucocorticoid (GC) therapy, there is a persisting concern that poor growth still exists. The mechanism of growth failure in children with IBD is multifactorial and includes poor nutrition, chronic inflammation, and the prolonged use of steroids. These factors interfere with growth through disturbance of the GH-IGF axis at the peripheral or central level. Growth improvement through manipulation of the GH-IGF axis may offer a therapeutic option which needs further exploration. Nonetheless, the assessment of prevalence of growth impairment in children receiving advanced therapy may be needed before launching studies of alternative forms of growth-promoting endocrine therapy.

Methods: The study is a retrospective analysis of growth and therapy data of 116 children with CD (mean age at diagnosis 10.8 years), at time of diagnosis (T0), at 1 (T1), 2 (T2) and 3 years (T3) after diagnosis and at maximum follow-up (MF).

Results: There was a significant reduction in mean height z-score (HtSDS) between T0 and T1. No significant difference was observed in HtSDS after that. Moreover, no change was observed in mean ΔHtSDS at T1, T2, T3 and MF. However, there was a significant increase in mean HVSDS (10th, 90th) from −1.4 (−7.4 to 7.4) to −0.6 (−7.5 to 6.1) between T1 and T2, from −0.6 to −0.1 between T2 and T3 and from −0.1 to 0.6 between T3 and MF. There was a negative association between HtSDS and the use of prednisolone, azathioprine, methotrexate and weight SDS. A negative association was also found between ΔHtSDS and use of prednisolone and a positive association between HVSDS with age and WtSDS.

Conclusion: The authors concluded that short stature and slow growth continue to be encountered in a subgroup of children with CD despite advances in therapy. They suggest that change in HtSDS may be a more robust parameter in children with chronic disease when there is a high prevalence of children of peripubertal age.

Comments   Although the majority of children with CD are not particularly short and there is an improvement in growth during the first year after diagnosis, this study provides clear evidence that despite advances in therapy, short stature and slow growth continue to be encountered in a subgroup of children with CD. The mean HtSDS of our population as well as the percentage of children with HtSDS <−2 were similar to those reported in other recent studies. Our observation that HtSDS did not improve in spite of significant improvement in HVSDS is similar to the findings in previous reports and may suggest that the reduction in growth deceleration, as reflected by improving HV, is not sufficient to improve overall height but simply prevents any further deterioration in height. Many studies of growth in children with a complex condition such as IBD explore the association between growth and disease factors, including drug therapy. The study highlights that investigation of such associations need a long follow-up as the choice and duration of therapy for IBD depends on the acute presentation and subsequent progress.

Overall Commentary: Over the last year a number of studies have evaluated growth impairment as well as the outcomes of therapeutic intervention aimed to improve growth in children with IBD. Given the persistent deficit in height in children with IBD, there is a need for further improvements in therapy that focus on growth. Clinicians and investigators need to pay more attention to puberty aspects, especially in this group of conditions which often present during the peripubertal period, since a substantial amount of growth occurs during puberty. It has been suggested that pubertal development and progress is not significantly affected in children with IBD treated with the current therapeutic modalities. It would, therefore, be useful to investigate whether growth during puberty is optimal or not. The studies that have been performed over the last year also highlight the large variation amongst investigators as to how they describe growth and pubertal progress. There is a need for greater consistency and harmony in reporting results. Finally, these studies cannot be performed without close collaboration between a multidisciplinary group of experts from fields that include anthropometry, endocrinology, nutrition medicine and gastroenterology.

Acknowledgements: M.A.A is funded by the Higher Education Ministry of Libyan Government. S.F.A is supported by the Chief Scientist Office of Scotland and ISPEN.

Cystic Fibrosis

Better nutritional status in early childhood is associated with improved clinical outcomes and survival in patients with cystic fibrosis

Yen EH[1], Quinton H[2], Borowitz D[3]

[1]Department of Pediatrics, Harvard Medical School, Division of Gastroenterology and Nutrition, Children's Hospital Boston, Boston, MA, USA; [2]Dartmouth Medical School, Lebanon, NH, USA; [3]Department of Pediatrics, State University of New York at Buffalo School of Medicine and Biomedical Sciences, Women and Children's Hospital of Buffalo, Buffalo, NY, USA

J Pediatr 2013; 162: 530–535.e1

Aims: The aim of the current study was to evaluate the impact of nutritional status early in life on the timing and velocity of height growth, lung function, complications of CF, and survival through age 18 years.

Methods: The study included the data extracted from the CFF Patient Registry for patients born between 1989 and 1992. The patients were stratified by peak weight-for-age percentile (WAP) at age 4–5 years into 4 groups: <10th percentile, 10th to <25th percentile, 25th to <50th percentile, and ≥50th percentile. Outcomes were assessed through 2009 at the age of 18 years and comparisons between height-for-age percentile (HAP), predicted forced expiratory volume in 1 s (FEV1)%, and survival were made across strata. Other outcomes included BMI, pulmonary exacerbations, cystic fibrosis-related diabetes mellitus (CFRD), *Pseudomonas aeruginosa* infection, and survival.

Results: The cohort consisted of 3,142 patients. On average, patients with CF who achieved a WAP >50% at age 4 years reached a much higher HAP early on in life and maintained their height advantage into adulthood over the group of patients with CF and a WAP <50% at age 4 years. This gain in HAP by WAP at age 4 years was incremental and was sustained throughout childhood, indicating a strong association between WAP at age 4 years and height throughout life. Each higher WAP group had incrementally better FEV1% predicted throughout the period of observation, but the greatest difference in FEV1% predicted occurred between the WAP <10% and 10–25%. The rate of decline in FEV1% predicted was similar across all WAP groups until age 18–19 years. There were 294 deaths during the observational period; cumulative survival over the whole follow-up period in the entire population was 91%. Survival was highest on average in patients with better nutritional status at age 4 years. Higher WAP and HAP at age 4 years predicted a higher rate of survival into adulthood (p < 0.0001). CF-related diabetes, acute exacerbations, and hospital days by age 18 years were also strongly associated with WAP at age 4 years.

Conclusions: Patients in the highest weight and height percentiles at age 4 years achieved better heights by 18 years, had fewer pulmonary exacerbations, spent fewer days in the hospital, and had improved survival.

Growth during puberty in cystic fibrosis: a retrospective evaluation of a French cohort

Bournez M[1], Bellis B[2], Huet F[1]

[1]Department of Paediatrics, University Hospital, Dijon, France; [2]National Institute of Demographic Studies, Paris, France

Arch Dis Child 2012; 97: 714–720

Aims: The primary outcome of the study was to assess the longitudinal growth pattern in a large cohort of French patients with CF and to determine the extent to which growth during puberty affects final height. In addition, the study aimed to explore the potential relationships between growth, nutritional status and respiratory function in children with CF.

Methods: The study included the data from the French CF registry collected between 1999 and 2004. Eight groups of patients aged 8–15 in 1999 were selected. Individual characteristics (age, height, weight) and lung function, evaluated by FEV1 were recorded. The means of individual heights in each age group were used to construct the height curves by sex.

Results: The study evaluated a sample of 729 children with CF among the 1,108 children born between 1984 and 1991 and followed by the registry from 1999 to 2004. For the 331 girls the height curve was very close to the median curve until the age of 12, when the curve descended to the –1 SD reference curve. The mean z-score of mean height was –0.32 at age 8 and –0.53 at 11 years. The z-score then decreased to a minimum of –0.88 at age 15, and remains under –0.50 after this age. The final height of 160.4 cm was reached at age 19, much later than the age of final height in the reference population which is attained at age 16. The age of pubertal onset was similar to the reference, but the peak height velocity (PHV), although occurring at the same age as in reference girls, was lower, and the pubertal spurt accounted for 16.7% (compared to 18.6% in healthy girls) of the final adult height. The mean height curve for boys (n = 389) showed normal growth until age 14, and then downgraded to the –1 SD of the reference curve. The final height in boys was reached at age 19, similar to the age of final height in healthy boys. The mean final height in boys with CF was less than that in the overall population (z-score –0.73). The age of pubertal onset was similar to that in reference boys (13 years), but the PHV was lower and the pubertal spurt accounted for 15.5% (18.4% in healthy boys) of the final height of CF boys. No correlations were found between BMI and PHV (r = 0.03, p = 0.71 in girls; r = 0.05, p = 0.44 in boys). No relationships were found either between lung function expressed by FEV1 and growth in boys (r = 0.09, p = 0.16), but there was a weak but significant positive relationship between growth and FEV1 (r = 0.17, p = 0.02) in girls.

Conclusions: The longitudinal follow-up of this French cohort of patients showed that the onset of puberty in children with CF was comparable to healthy children, but PHV was decreased and contributed less to the final adult height. The final height was significantly lower than that in the reference population, even though it remained within the normal range. Growth and lung function were not correlated in boys, however there was a weak but significant correlation between lung function and growth in girls, which might be explained by the greater rest energy expenditure in girls than in boys after the pubertal spurt.

Pubertal height velocity and associations with prepubertal and adult heights in cystic fibrosis

Zhang Z[1], Lindstrom MJ[2], Lai HJ[1,2,3]

[1]Departments of Nutritional Sciences, [2]Biostatistics and Medical Informatics, and [3]Pediatrics, University of Wisconsin-Madison, Madison, WI, USA

J Pediatr 2013; 163: 376–382.e1

Aims: Using the US CFF Registry data of patients' anthropometry and follow-up the authors evaluated the relationship between prepubertal and pubertal growth velocity (timing and magnitude) and final adult height in children with CF.

Methods: Using height measurements, the authors constructed puberty height velocity (PHV) curves for CF patients. Using longitudinal standards of PHV for healthy North American children developed by Tanner and Davies, PHV was classified into normal (PHV neither delayed nor attenuated), delayed (PHV delayed but not attenuated), attenuated (PHV attenuated but not delayed), and delayed and attenuated. CF phenotypes, prepubertal nutritional status and genetic height potential were introduced as variables.

Results: Of the 4,198 individuals with CF born in 1984–1987, 309 died, 951 were lost to follow-up before age 18 years, and 1,076 had <3 height measurements per year during age 10–18 years, leaving 1,862 patients to include in the study. PHV in children with CF occurred later (0.5 years later in boys and 0.6 years later in girls) and showed reduced magnitude (1.1 cm less in boys and 1.3 cm in girls). Results from fitting individual curves revealed that PHV was normal in 60.3%, delayed in 9.4%, attenuated in 20.8%, and delayed and attenuated in 5.3%. In the remaining 4.2%, PHV could not be ascertained. More boys had normal PHV than girls, p = 0.002. PHV magnitude and total gain from height take-off at puberty was different and depended on whether the puberty was delayed and/or attenuated. Considering parental height, 80% of boys with CF and 77% of girls with CF had adult heights below their average parental height percentiles. Multivariate analyses revealed PHV age, PHV magnitude, and prepubertal height at age 7 years were stronger predictors of adult height (all with p < 0.001). Specifically, later PHV was associated with smaller magnitude of PHV but greater adult height. Larger PHV magnitude was associated with greater adult height after adjusting for PHV age.

Conclusions: Using a novel, semi-parametric growth curve model, this study showed that 23% of boys with CF and 30% of girls with CF had impaired PHV magnitude that was below the 5th percentile of healthy children. Besides that, children with CF born in the mid-1980s experienced delayed pubertal PHV compared with healthy children and had lower final height, as the majority (80% of boys and 70% of girls) did not reach their genetic potential. Prepubertal height at age 7 years was found to be a strong determinant of adult height in both sexes. Since the greatest likelihood of achieving optimal growth at age 6 years is through maximizing weight gain during the first years of life, this study further emphasize the importance of maintaining adequate growth through pre-adolescence.

Longitudinal trends in nutritional status and the relation between lung function and BMI in cystic fibrosis: a population-based cohort study

Stephenson AL[1-4], Mannik LA[1], Walsh S[1], Brotherwood M[1], Robert R[1], Darling PB[2,4], Nisenbaum R[2,4], Moerman J[3], Stanojevic S[3,4]

[1]The Adult Cystic Fibrosis Program, St. Michael's Hospital, Toronto, ON, Canada; [2]The Keenan Research Centre in the Li Ka Shing Knowledge Institute of St. Michael's Hospital, Toronto, ON, Canada; [3]The Research Institute, The Hospital for Sick Children, Toronto, ON, Canada; [4]Departments of Medicine and Nutritional Sciences and Institute of Health Policy, Management, and Evaluation, Dalla Lana School of Public Health, University of Toronto, Toronto, ON, Canada

Am J Clin Nutr 2013; 97: 872–877

Aims: The aim of the present study was to investigate the nutritional status evolution during a long-term follow-up of a CF cohort followed at the Adult CF Clinic in Toronto.

Methods: The study examined nutritional status assessed as WHO BMI and the relationship between BMI and lung function in 909 individuals with CF. FEV1 expressed as a percentage of the normal predicted values for height and sex (FEV1% predicted), height and weight were measured at every clinic visit. The subjects were classified in 4 cohorts based of birth year (<1960, 1960–1969, 1970–1979, >1979) and the BMI was parted according to the year the clinical measurements were taken (<1990, 1991–1999, >2000). Due to the skewed distribution of BMI and age, these variables were log transformed.

Results: The study cohort study included 909 individuals followed from 1985 to 2011. The average BMI increased from 20.7 ± 2.7 before 1990 to 22.3 ± 3.4 in the most recent decade (2000–2011). The proportion of underweight individuals has also decreased from 20.6% before 1990 to 11.1% in the most recent decade. The proportion of adequate-weight subjects slightly decreased (72.4% in 1980s, 72.6% in the 1990s, to 70.5% in the 2000s), whereas the proportion of overweight/obese subjects increased from 7.0% in the 1980s to 15.8% in the 1990s and to 18.4% in the most recent cohort (p trend <0.001). Multivariable models showed that, overall, BMI increased by 0.4%/year from 1985 to 2011. The rate of BMI increase in PS subjects was much greater than in PI subjects (3.8% compared with 0.4%/year, respectively; p < 0.001). The BMI of 651 individuals evaluated between 2000 and 2011 showed that 17% of CF subjects were underweight, 60% had adequate weight, 18% were overweight, and 3.8% were obese. After adjustment for age, height, sex, CFRD, pancreatic status, and birth cohort, lung function showed improvement as BMI increased. The magnitude of FEV1 improvement was different across BMI categories: in the underweight group, a 10% increase in BMI resulted in a 4% relative increase in FEV1, in the subjects within adequate range BMI there was a 5% relative increase in FEV1, and in those overweight there was a 2% increase in FEV1. On average, FEV1 decreased at a rate of 1%/year, and there were no significant differences in the rate of FEV1 decline in the three BMI categories. Other significant independent predictors of FEV1, identified in the multivariable model, included age [older age was associated with lower FEV1% (predicted; p < 0.001), pancreatic status (PS subjects had higher FEV1% predicted), and the presence of CFRD (CFRD subjects had lower FEV1% predicted].

Conclusion: This longitudinal, population-based cohort showed a significant shift over a 25-year period in the distribution of BMI in adults with CF. Within a contemporary cohort of individuals with CF, fewer individuals were malnourished and more individuals were overweight compared with 20 years earlier. The study showed that improvements in nutritional status were associated with improvements in lung function which was better in the average BMI subgroup of the CF population.

Stunting is an independent predictor of mortality in patients with cystic fibrosis

Vieni G[1,2], Faraci S[2], Collura M[3], Lombardo M[2], Traverso G[3], Cristadoro S[2], Termini L[3], Lucanto MC[2], Furnari ML[3], Trimarchi G[4], Triglia MR[2], Costa S[1,2], Pellegrino S[1,2], Magazzù G[2]

[1]Clinical and Biomolecular Hepato-Gastroenterology of Pediatric and Adult Age, University Hospital 'G. Martino', Messina Italy; [2]Pediatric Gastroenterology and Cystic Fibrosis Unit, University Hospital 'G. Martino', Messina Italy; [3]Cystic Fibrosis Regional Centre, 2nd Pediatric Unit, Children's Hospital 'Di Cristina', Palermo, Italy; [4]Department of Statistics, University of Messina, Messina, Italy

Clin Nutr 2013; 32: 382–385

Aims: The relationship between nutritional status and survival in patients with CF has been much studied. This study aim was to evaluate the relationship between stunting (as a measure of chronic malnutrition) and mortality in a nested case-control CF population cohort.

Methods: This retrospective case-control study included a cohort of 393 CF patients older than 6 years of age, 193 pediatric (less than 18 years) and 200 adult patients followed at the CF Regional Center in Palermo and at the Satellite Center in Messina through December 2007. The study cases included 95 patients who died, 47 children and 48 adults. The controls were 298 alive patients, 146 younger and 152 older than 18 years. Short stature (stunting) was defined by a height <5th percentile. Body wasting was defined by a body mass index (BMI) <10th percentile in pediatric patients, and <18.5 in adult patients.

Results: The prevalence of stunting was 24.4%, similar in males and females (24.5 and 24.3%, respectively). The prevalence of wasting was 35.3%; not significantly higher in females than in males (38.3 and 32.3%, respectively). In the multivariate analysis, stunting, body wasting, and FEV1 significantly predict the risk of mortality. Stunting (OR 2.22; 95% CI 1.10–4.46), wasting (OR 5.27; 95% CI 2.66–10.41), and FEV1 <40% of predicted (OR 10.60; 95% CI 5.43–20.67) increased the risk of death in this cohort.

Conclusions: In this study, stunting, wasting and FEV1 were independently predictors of mortality risk.

Use of body mass index percentile to identify fat-free mass depletion in children with cystic fibrosis

Engelen MP[1], Schroder R[1], Van der Hoorn K[1], Deutz NE[1], Com G[2]

[1]Center for Translational Research in Aging and Longevity, Donald W. Reynolds Institute on Aging, University of Arkansas for Medical Sciences, Little Rock, AR, USA; [2]Pediatric Pulmonology, University of Arkansas for Medical Sciences and Arkansas Children's Hospital, Little Rock, AR, USA

Clin Nutr 2012; 31: 927–933

Aims: The study aimed to evaluate: (1) the prevalence of underweight [diagnosed by body mass index (BMI) percentile] and free fat mass (FFM) depletion, (2) the association of FFM depletion with changes in body composition and increased morbidity (reduced lung function, loss of bone mineral density), and (3) use of BMI percentiles as predictors of FFM depletion and morbidity.

Methods: 77 children, aged 8–21 years, with CF were evaluated in this retrospective study. Height and weight were obtained and BMI percentiles calculated. Fat-free mass (FFM), fat mass (FM), bone mineral content (BMC) and density (BMD) were obtained by dual-energy x-ray absorptiometry (DXA).

Results: 24 children (31%) were malnourished, as defined by the FFMI and/or BMI% criteria; 16% had low BMI% and low FFMI; 14% had normal BMI and low FFMI (hidden depletion), and 1% had low BMI% and normal FFMI. Overall, 30% of patients were characterized by FFM depletion. The sensitivity of BMI% for detecting FFM depletion was 52% and the specificity was 98%. BMC (percentage of normative data) was reduced in the group with low BMI% and FFMI (p < 0.001) and in the hidden FFMI depletion group (p < 0.05) as compared to the normal BMI% and FFMI group. BMD of the whole-body and spine z-score were lower (p < 0.01) in those with low BMI% and FFM as compared to normal BMI% and FFM. Below the 20th BMI% the percentage of patients with a BMD z-score <−1 SD increased steeply whereas no differences were found in the percentage of patients with a reduced BMD in the 20–49th BMI% group. FEV1 and forced vital capacity (FVC) were reduced in both the hidden FFM depletion group (p < 0.05) and the low BMI% and FFM group (p < 0.01). FEV1 was significantly correlated with FFM (% norm, r = 0.39, p < 0.001) and FM (% norm, r = 0.30, p < 0.01) but not with FM/FFM (r = 0.21). With the decline in BMI%, there was also a gradual reduction in mean FEV1. Below the 20th BMI%, mean FEV1 dropped below 80% predicted, a threshold for abnormal lung function in children with CF. Investigation of the BMI% cut-off point that would predict FFM depletion and poor clinical outcome showed a gradual reduction in FFM% with the decline in BMI%. Below the 20th BMI%, there was a drop in FFM% below 90% of normative values which corresponds to FFMI <5th percentile. 57% of the patients in the 10–20th BMI% group had FFM depletion, compared to 18% in the 20–30th BMI% group. Nearly all patients (92%) with BMI% <10 were FFM depleted.

Conclusions: FFM depletion in children with CF is prevalent and is poorly detected when using the 10% BMI cut-off, indicating that a large share of patients with hidden FFM depletion would have been missed when malnutrition was defined only by these criteria. Low FFM values were associated with reduced lung function and bone mineral loss indicating the clinical importance of measuring body composition in children with CF.

Genetic modifiers of nutritional status in cystic fibrosis

Bradley GM[1], Blackman SM[1], Watson CP[2], Doshi VK[2], Cutting GR[1,2]

[1]Department of Pediatrics, Johns Hopkins University, Baltimore, MD, USA; [2]McKusick-Nathans Institute of Genetic Medicine, Johns Hopkins University, Baltimore, MD, USA

Am J Clin Nutr 2012; 96: 1299–1308

Aims: The study investigated the influence of modifier genes on nutritional status of children with CF.

Methods: Longitudinal height and weight data were collected from 2000 to 2010 from the CF Twin-Sibling Study. Family members all shared the same CFTR genotype. BMI and z-scores for weight and height were calculated. A phenotype was derived by calculating the average-per-quarter BMI z-scores from 5 to 10 years of age (BMI_{z5to10}). Sex, birth cohort, age at CF diagnosis, diagnosis by newborns' screening, F508del homozygosity, pancreatic insufficiency (PI), history of meconium ileus (MI), presence of a gastrostomy, FEV_{q6to10}, and insurance type were evaluated for their contributions to variability in BMI_{z5to10}.

Results: Longitudinal height and weight data were collected for 1,124 subjects (130 monozygous twins and 952 siblings) with CF from 800 families. The median height z-score for all included subjects was –0.58 (range –4.61 to 2.46), which corresponded to the 28th CDC percentile; the median weight z-score was –0.42 (range –6.23 to 2.38), which corresponded to the 34th CDC percentile. The median BMI z-score was –0.07 (range –3.89 to 2.30), which corresponded to the 47th CDC percentile. There were no significant differences in the average BMI z-score between monozygous twins and siblings and dizygous twins and siblings. All covariates in the model remained independent predictors of BMI-$_{z5to10}$ in the multivariate models. Adjusted BMI z-score phenotypes were generated for female sex, birth cohort, PI, and history of MI (BMI-$_{zadj}$) and in a second analysis for BMI-$_{zadj}$ plus for FEV$_{q6to10}$ (BMI-$_{zadjFEV}$), which considered the influence of lung function on BMI for subsequent heritability and linkage analyses. There was a high degree of concordance for BMI in individuals who shared 100% of genes, for monozygous twins (0.80–0.85 for 58–65 pairs). The dizygous twin-only groups had lower correlation coefficients (0.58–0.66 for 21 dizygous twin pairs; 0.41–0.57 for 13 same-sex, dizygous twin pairs), which indicated a lower concordance in this group of twins who shared, on average, 50% of genes. Correlation coefficients for the dizygous twin and sibling group were 0.5 (0.25–0.31 for 122–148 pairs). Linkage results for individuals with PI (BMI-$_{zadj-PI}$; 358 sibling pairs) revealed 2 prominent genome-wide significant peaks on chromosomes 1p36.1 (LOD: 5.3) and 5q14 (LOD: 5.1). Restriction of the analysis to the 219 sibling pairs who were homozygous for the F508del mutation (BMI-$_{zadj-F508del}$) preserved the peak on chromosome 1p36.1 (LOD: 4.6) but decreased the evidence for linkage on chromosome 5q14 (LOD: 3.4). Adjustment of BMI for lung function (BMI-$_{zadjFEV-PI}$; 350 sibling pairs) decreased the LOD score for the locus on chromosome 1p36.1 (LOD: 3.4) but increased the evidence for linkage at an adjacent region from chromosome 1p31–22 (LOD: 2.4); linkage on chromosome 5q14 (LOD: 5.2) was unaffected. Quantitative trait locus (QTL) heritability at 1p36.1 and 5q14 after correction for potential bias represented ≥16% and ≥15% of the BMI variance.

Conclusions: This is the first study on the nutritional status of young twins and siblings with CF which shows that genes other than CFTR influence the variation in BMI. Specifically, the results from this study suggested that modifier genes located at the 1p36.1 locus influence both nutritional status and lung function, whereas chromosome 5q14 encompasses a gene that modifies nutritional status that is independent of lung disease severity.

Oral calorie supplements for cystic fibrosis

Smyth RL[1], Walters S[2]

[1]Institute of Child Health, UCL, London, UK; [2]c/o CFGD Group, Institute of Child Health, University of Liverpool, Liverpool, UK

Cochrane Database Syst Rev 2012; 10: CD000406

Aims: This Cochrane systematic review aimed to evaluate the benefits of dietary advice or oral nutritional supplementations for at least 1 month in patients with CF on different outcomes, i.e. weight gain and growth, body composition (primary outcomes), lung function, gastrointestinal adverse effects or activity levels (secondary outcomes).

Methods: The authors searched the Cochrane CF Trials Register for randomized or quasi-randomized controlled trials which compared the use of oral calorie supplements to increase caloric intake with no specific intervention.

Results: The literature search identified 21 trials. Only three trials (131 patients) fulfilled the inclusion criteria [3–5] and were included in the final meta-analysis. There was no significant difference between the groups at any time point with regard to change in weight, weight percentile, height,

height percentile, weight for height or body mass index (BMI) (primary outcomes). There were no differences between intervention (oral supplementation) and non-intervention groups with regard to secondary outcomes including total (oral or supplemented) intake of calories, protein, fat, feeding behavior or measures of quality of life. Forced expiratory volume in 1 s (FEV1) (% predicted) was significantly decreased at 3 months in the control group but not at 6 and 12 months. The change in forced vital capacity (FVC) (reported only by Poustie et al. [5]), was not significantly different between groups at 3, 6 or 12 months. The single study [5] that evaluated the presence of adverse effects of oral supplements reported no differences on diarrhea, appetite, abdominal bloating, episodes of distal intestinal obstruction syndrome and any other adverse effects between intervention and non-intervention groups.

Conclusions: This systematic review showed that short-term use of oral supplements did not improve the nutritional status in children with CF and mild to moderate malnutrition. Since no difference in nutritional status or lung function was reported with the use of oral nutrition supplements, one may conclude that dietary advice alone is also a satisfactory approach to the management of people with CF and moderate malnutrition. This systematic review raises questions about the utility of the practice of prescribing oral nutrition supplements for the nutritional care and rehabilitation of children with CF.

Nutritional outcomes following gastrostomy in children with cystic fibrosis

Bradley GM[1], Carson KA[2], Leonard AR[1], Mogayzel PJ Jr[3], Oliva-Hemker M[1]

[1]Division of Pediatric Gastroenterology and Nutrition, Johns Hopkins University School of Medicine, Baltimore, MD, USA; [2]Department of Epidemiology, Johns Hopkins Bloomberg School of Public Health, Baltimore, MD, USA; [3]Eudowood Division of Pediatric Respiratory Sciences, Johns Hopkins University School of Medicine, Baltimore, MD, USA

Pediatr Pulmonol 2012; 47: 743–748

Aims: The primary aim of the study was to evaluate the ability of nutrient supplementation using a gastrostomy tube (GT) to improve nutritional status in children with CF and low BMI. Furthermore, the study evaluated the effects of GT placement and supplemental nutrition on lung function, number of hospitalizations for pulmonary exacerbation and complications during and after GT placement.

Methods: This retrospective study evaluated 40 patients (20 children with GT and 20 controls) 2–20 years old with data at least 1 year after GT placement. Each one of the 'cases' (children with GT) was pair-matched with a child with CF who did not have a GT ('controls'). The cases and controls were matched for age ± 2.5 years, sex, pancreatic status, BMI percentile ± 10% and, when available, FEV1 ± 20%. Data on GT placement technique, complications during and after GT placement and nutritional supplementation through GT were collected in the 'cases' group. For the controls, use of oral nutritional supplementation, appetite stimulant and/or a gastroenterology (GI) referral for GT placement at any time during the 1-year follow-up period were recorded. Nutritional and lung function data (including height, weight, BMI, and percent predicted FEV1) were obtained at the enrollment visit, 6-month (±3 months) and 1-year (±3 months) follow-up. The number of hospitalizations required for pulmonary exacerbation during the 1-year follow-up period was also recorded.

Results: GT placement was without complications in 15/20 and whole protein formula was given to 18/20 children. GT delivered about 50% of the 110–200% dietary reference intake recommendation. The whole GT supplementation was delivered continuously overnight. A dose of pancreatic enzymes was given at the beginning and the end of the feeds. At the 6-month follow-up visit, 7 (35%) of the cases and 1 (5%) of the controls reached BMI ≥50th percentile (p < 0.04). The patients supplemented by GT were almost 10 times as likely to reach BMI ≥50th percentile at 6 months compared to the control group (OR = 9.70; 95% CI 1.05–484.7). At 1-year follow-up, 8 (40%) of the cases and 3 (15%) of the controls had reached BMI ≥50th percentile (p < 0.16) (OR = 3.65; 95% CI 0.69–25.86). The mean ± SD BMI was significantly better compared to controls (p < 0.001) at 6 months, but not at 12 months. The mean weight z-score improved significantly from the baseline compared to controls at 6 months (p < 0.001) and 12 months (p < 0.01) but the change in mean height z-score was comparable between cases and controls. At 6 months, the mean ± SD BMI and mean weight z-score in the GT group improved from the baseline compared to controls (p < 0.001), while there was no difference in mean height z-score between the two groups. At 1 year, the cases still had a higher mean BMI z-score than the controls, but the difference from baseline no longer achieved statistical significance. The change in mean weight z-score was still statistically significant (p < 0.01), but the change in mean height z-score was again comparable. The groups were similar in the change in mean predicted FEV1 from baseline to 6 and 12 months and there were no statistically significant differences between the cases and controls in the number of hospitalizations required for pulmonary exacerbation. By 1 year, 1 child was no longer receiving supplemental nutrition via the GT. At 1 year, 12/20 controls were advised to take oral supplements and 6 were prescribed an appetite stimulant. One patient was referred for GT placement.

Conclusions: In this retrospective study, nutritional support using supplemental feedings via a GT was shown to improve weight gain in patients with CF. According to the current study, children with CF who had a BMI <50th percentile for age and received a GT were almost 10 times as likely to reach BMI ≥50th percentile at 6 months compared to matched patients who did not receive a GT and were 3.65 times as likely to reach BMI ≥50th percentile by 12 months. The conclusions are weakened by the fact that these changes did not reach statistical significance.

Recombinant growth hormone therapy for cystic fibrosis in children and young adults

Thaker V[1], Haagensen AL[2], Carter B[3], Fedorowicz Z[4], Houston BW[5]

[1]Haverstraw Pediatrics, Haverstraw, NY, USA; [2]Children's Hospital Boston, Boston, MA, USA; [3]Cancer Research UK Clinical Trials Unit, School of Cancer Sciences, Birmingham University, Birmingham, UK; [4]The Cochrane Collaboration (UKCC), Awali, Bahrain; [5]School of Health & Social Care, Teesside University, Middlesbrough, UK

Cochrane Database Syst Rev 2013; 6: CD008901

Aims: The study aimed to review the evidence on the effectiveness and safety of recombinant human growth hormone (rhGH) therapy in improving lung function, quality of life and clinical status of children and young adults with CF.

Methods: This is a systematic review of all the randomized controlled trials (RCT) trials that reported the results of rhGH treatment in children and adolescents with CF.

Results: The authors identified 22 potentially eligible studies for further evaluation. Only four studies (161 participants) were included in the final review. Two of the studies were RCT of parallel design [6, 7]. One was a cross-over study with two periods of treatment [8] and one study was quasi-randomized [9]. Three studies used rhGH in a standard dose of approximately 0.3 mg/kg/week compared with no treatment; one study had three treatment arms: placebo, standard dose (0.3 mg/kg/week) and high dose (0.5 mg/kg/week). Pulmonary function reported as FEV1 or FVC [6] showed no evidence of an effect from rhGH treatment. Height and weight were not significantly changed by rhGH treatment [9], but height velocity showed a significant difference in favor of rhGH, MD 2.10 (95% CI 0.54–3.66). Fasting blood glucose at 6 months [6] showed a significant increase in the rhGH treatment group, MD 12.40 (95% CI 3.76–21.04), however the difference in postprandial glucose levels was not significant, MD 12.10 mg/dl (95% CI –7.18 to 31.38) (0.54–3.66). Muscle strength and the number of pulmonary exacerbations were also no different in the rhGH treatment.

Conclusions: rhGH treatment in children with CF achieved modest improvements in anthropometric measures (height, weight, height and weight velocity and lean tissue mass). At this stage, the question of whether this improvement translates into better pulmonary outcomes, reduction in morbidity and improved quality of life has not been answered from the available evidence, due to scarcity of data.

Comments   Cystic fibrosis (CF) is a common autosomal recessive genetic disorder, diagnosed in approximately 1 in 2,500 births, more often in populations of Caucasian descent. The gene, the CF transmembrane regulator (CFTR) located on chromosome 7, encodes a protein that functions as a cAMP-regulated chloride channel and controls the flow of sodium and chloride ions across the cell membrane. Most patients with CF (85%) carry mutations which are associated with pancreatic insufficiency. The clinical features of CF can be highly variable, including non-specific respiratory symptoms or gastrointestinal symptoms and malnutrition. In the past, growth failure and weight loss were seen as inevitable in the face of progressive lung disease.

In 1988, Corey et al. [10] reported growth, pulmonary function and survival in 499 CF patients from Boston (USA) and 534 from Toronto (Canada) followed from 1972 to 1981. Although patients' characteristics were comparable in the two populations, height and weight percentiles were higher in patients from Toronto than in Boston and also their survival (30 vs. 21 years). The only difference was that Canadian patients had a better nutritional status resulting from a non-restricted dietary fat diet and the use of coated pancreatic enzymes. Since that report, many studies have shown that nutritional status during childhood is the most important single factor determining pulmonary status (and hence likely survival) in CF individuals.

In order to achieve the most favorable outcomes, the care of children with CF should address both nutritional status and lung function. Normal growth, therefore, has been decreed by Cystic Fibrosis Foundation (CFF) as the key goal of nutritional support in children with CF [11]. Nutritional status by all parameters (wasting, stunting, body composition) has been shown to affect lung function and survival in patients with CF in many studies before and this year too (cf. Yen et al., Bournez et al., Zhang et al., Stephenson et al., Vieni et al.).

As children get older, the nutrient requirements increase, but progression of lung disease compromises nutritional status by increasing daily energy demands, interfering with appetite, and resulting in a decreased overall energy intake. Many studies have shown that growth deviation takes place during the puberty years as patients with CF have delayed puberty and diminished growth pubertal spurt (cf. Zhang et al., Bournez et al.). This maturational delay affects negatively final adult height, as 70–80% of children with CF did not reach their genetic potential. Growth delay and deficit do not affect only the final adult height but also survival, as shown in the study by Vieni et al.

Evaluation of nutritional intake and growth must be made at every visit. Every effort should be made to maintain ideal body weight (IBW%) in children <2 years (>95%) and BMI in children >2 years (ideally >50th percentile). BMI is an easy, quick, safe, and low-cost method that is considered the gold standard to approach nutritional status in children with CF >2 years. Data from the CFF Registry has consistently demonstrated a positive association between BMI and lung function. Several studies have also explored the relationship between BMI and lean muscle mass and measures of disease severity in CF. Engelen et al. have shown that FFM depletion is prevalent and not always detected using BMI%, furthermore, FFM was correlated with FEV1 (a measure of lung function).

Using the data from CF Twin-Sibling Study and Cystic Fibrosis Foundation Patient Registry, the original study of Bradley et al. had evaluated the relative contribution of genetic modifiers to the nutritional status of young children with CF. Linkage analyses pointed that genes on chromosomes 1 and 5 significantly influence the BMI variation in children with CF. The search for CF-modifying genes represents the opportunity to further insight into the pathophysiology of malnutrition in children with CF and discovery of potential new targets for nutritional intervention.

There is evidence that nutritional support can delay the decline in lung function, translating into improved health, quality of life, and length of survival in these patients. Studies in the early 1980s, which reported positive effects of dietary counseling and/or supplements, were however conducted in patients who had been placed on a low-fat diet before the study. The recent Cochrane systematic review (cf. Smyth and Walters), however, reported no improvement in nutritional parameters or pulmonary function in children with CF on oral nutritional supplements. Enteral tube feeding, using gastrostomy, usually delivered as overnight feeds with appropriate enzyme therapy, may provide approximately 30–50% of estimated daily energy requirements. Supplemental gastrostomy feedings were shown to be associated with improvements in weight and height percentiles for age, increases in percent of body fat and fat-free mass and sustained growth. The retrospective study of Bradley et al. however reported no effect on pulmonary function status or disease severity (hospitalizations). Currently, most studies on supplemental gastrostomy feedings are, however, retrospective and since randomization is not feasible/ethical, only cohort longitudinal studies at best will be expected.

Use of rhGH for the treatment of growth deficit as well as an anabolic agent has been addressed by several studies. A systematic review published in 2010 which evaluated 10 controlled clinical trials and 8 observational studies showed that in the controlled trials, markers of pulmonary function, anthropometrics, and bone mineralization appeared to be increased compared with controls [12]. With regard to long-term health issues, such as pulmonary exacerbations, hospitalizations, or mortality, the only significant finding was that GH therapy seemed to reduce the rate of hospitalizations. The recent Cochrane systematic review (cf. Thaker et al.) which included 4 RCTs found only modest improvements in anthropometric measures (height, weight, height and weight velocity and lean tissue mass) but no evidence of better pulmonary function, reduced morbidity or improved quality of life.

According to CFF nutrition consensus, children and adolescents with CF are expected to experience typical growth when appropriate nutrition and pancreatic enzyme replacement therapy are provided. In 2008, nutritional recommendations for infants and children with CF provided evidence-based and consensus recommendations for many aspects of nutrition in CF patients [3]. Unfortunately, good quality evidence to support precise nutrition recommendations for patients with CF is missing, although efforts have been made to use available evidence to set care standards. Moreover, the benefit of providing invasive nutrition besides improving the patient's nutritional status and growth is questionable in terms of survival and lung function. In general, awareness of clinic staff about the overall nutritional status of their patient population and timely nutritional support when clinical indices fall below standards should be standard of care [13].

Cerebral Palsy

Energy requirements in preschool-age children with cerebral palsy

Walker JL[1,2], Bell KL[1-4], Boyd RN[2-4], Davies PSW[1]

[1]Children's Nutrition Research Centre, School of Medicine, The University of Queensland, Brisbane, QLD, Australia; [2]The Queensland Cerebral Palsy and Rehabilitation Research Centre, School of Medicine, The University of Queensland, Brisbane, QLD, Australia; [3]The Queensland Children's Medical Research Institute, The University of Queensland, Brisbane, QLD, Australia; [4]The Queensland Paediatric Rehabilitation Service, Royal Children's Hospital, Brisbane, QLD, Queensland, Australia

Am J Clin Nutr 2012; 96: 1309–1315

Aims: The study aimed to evaluate the energy requirements (ER) in a group of children with cerebral palsy (CP) using the doubly labeled water (DLW) method. The authors compared measured ER among children with CP and different functional abilities or motor dysfunction with typically developing children (TDC) and published estimation equations.

Methods: The study enrolled and evaluated 32 children with CP and 16 typically developed children (TDC) aged 2.9–4.4 years. Children with disorders or children on medications known to affect growth or metabolism were excluded from the study. Each child was given a dose of oxygen-18 and deuterium water (1.25 g/kg 10% $H_2{}^{18}O$ and 0.05 g/kg 99.8% $2H_2O$). A single urine sample was collected at baseline, daily urine samples were examined thereafter for 10 days. The production rate of carbon dioxide was calculated as the difference between the elimination rates of deuterium and oxygen-18 in conjunction with their dilution space. Oxygen consumption was determined by assuming a respiratory quotient of 0.85, and TEE was calculated using Weir equation [14]. Anthropometric measurements included weight, height/length/knee height. Functional ability (Gross Motor Function Classification System – GMFCS) and motor dysfunction type and distribution were evaluated using internationally accepted and validated criteria and classifications.

Results: The children with CP were shorter, lighter, and had lower free-fat mass indexes (FFMIs) than did the TDC ($p < 0.01$). Mean height z-scores and FFMI for children with CP decreased as ambulatory status declined ($p < 0.05$). Children with CP had significantly lower energy requirements (ERs) than did TDC [$p < 0.001$; mean difference (MD) = 1212kJ/d]. Ambulant CP children had, on average, an ER that was 16% lower than that of TDC. Marginally ambulant and non-ambulant children had an ER that was 31% lower than that of TDC and 18% lower than that of ambulant CP children. No statistical difference in ERs was found between ambulant children and TDC. The difference in GMFCS were responsible for 67% of the variability in ER ($r^2 = 0.67$). The FFM of the children contributed most to ERs variability. Correlation analyses of variables known to contribute to ERs showed that ERs were strongly positively correlated with FFM, weight, and height. When the influence of functional ability in the children with CP was considered, ERs decreased with increasing severity of disability (marginally ambulant and non-ambulant children had lower ER than did ambulant children). The estimated ERs from Rieken et al. [15] models were significantly less than the measured ER values, with a consistent bias of −1089kJ, representing an underestimation in ERs in the current population of 22%.

Conclusions: The results of this study confirm that ER recommendations, equations and energy intakes of typically developed children are not valid for use in children with CP, especially in more affected children. Motor disability (ambulation vs. non-ambulation) and FFM explained about 67% of the variability in ERs in this group of children with CP.

Validation of a modified three-day weighed food record for measuring energy intake in preschool-aged children with cerebral palsy

Walker JL[1,3,4], Bell KL[2-6], Boyd RN[2,4,5], Davies PS[1,3]

[1]Children's Nutrition Research Centre, UQ Department of Paediatrics and Child Health, Royal Children's Hospital, Herston, QLD, Australia; [2]Queensland Cerebral Palsy and Rehabilitation Research Centre, Department of Paediatrics and Child Health, The University of Queensland, Royal Brisbane Hospital, Herston, QLD, Australia; [3]Children's Nutrition Research Centre, School of Medicine, The University of Queensland, Brisbane, QLD, Australia; [4]Queensland Cerebral Palsy and Rehabilitation Research Centre, School of Medicine, The University of Queensland, Brisbane, QLD, Australia; [5]Queensland Children's Medical Research Institute, The University of Queensland, Brisbane, QLD, Australia; [6]Department of Paediatric Rehabilitation, Royal Children's Hospital, Brisbane, QLD, Queensland, Australia

Clin Nutr 2013; 32: 426–431

Aims: The aim of the current study was to validate the use of a modified 3-day weighed food record for measuring energy intake (EI) in a population of young children with CP.

Methods: The study included children aged between 35 and 54 months with a diagnosis of CP living in the community in the State of Queensland, Australia, and compared them to typically developing children (TDC) in the same age range residing in the same area. The children underwent the following evaluations: anthropometry measurements, functional ability using the Gross Motor Function Classification System (GMFCS) [16], energy assessment by a 3-day weighed food record, total energy expenditure (TEE) using the doubly labeled water (DLW) technique and oral motor and swallowing skills rating using the Feeding and Swallowing Competency Subset of the Dysphagia Disorders Survey for Paediatrics [17]. Validation of the 3-day weighed food record was done by comparing reported EI to measures of TEE for each individual child over the 10-day data collection period and the difference between reported EI and measured TEE (when expressed as a percentage of TEE) was less than 19%, an EI/TEE ratio of 1.00 indicating perfect reporting.

Results: The study population included 31 children (61% male) with CP aged from 2.9 to 4.4 years and 15 TDC (63% male) aged from 3.0 to 4.5 years. 13 children (42%) had moderate to severe feeding problems and 11/13 of these children were classified as GMFCS III, IV or V. Six children (19%) were tube-fed, all classified as GMFCS level V. In general, children with CP were shorter and lighter than the TDC. EI was statistically significantly less than TEE values for the children with CP as a total population and for the TDC [4,628 ± 1,325 vs. 5,142 ± 1,265 kJ/day (p < 0.01) in CP children and 5,310 ± 864 vs. 6,397 ± 779 kJ/day (p < 0.01) in TDC]. Evaluation of the EI as a percentage of

TEE for each group showed that children with moderate to severe CP had the most accurate reporting with a result of 4.3%. On average, 75% of the children with CP had EI results that were within 20% of their TEE values. The study showed no substantial overreporting as reported in previous literature. Considering functional ability, in children with moderate to severe CP the ratio of EI/TEE was 0.96 indicating greater accuracy compared to the TDC (0.83). Considering the influence of feeding method on the accuracy of reporting showed that orally-fed children displayed more accurate reporting when compared to those who were tube-fed, evidenced by a very low EI/TEE ratio of 1.01 indicating nearly perfect reporting.

Conclusions: Evaluation of 3-day weighed food record for assessment of energy intake in children with CP is a valid tool in pre-schoolchildren with CP among all the levels of functional ability and feeding difficulties or methods. The findings from this study are in contrast to previous literature reported by Stallings et al. [18] that reported gross overestimation of EI in school-aged children with CP.

The use of bioelectrical impedance analysis to estimate total body water in young children with cerebral palsy

Bell KL[1–4], Boyd RN[1,2], Walker JL[1,3], Stevenson RD[5], Davies PS[3]

[1]Queensland Cerebral Palsy and Rehabilitation Research Centre, School of Medicine, The University of Queensland, Brisbane, QLD, Australia; [2]Department of Paediatric Rehabilitation, Royal Children's Hospital, Brisbane, QLD, Australia; [3]Children's Nutrition Research Centre, School of Medicine, The University of Queensland, Brisbane, QLD, Australia; [4]Queensland Children's Medical Research Institute, The University of Queensland, Herston, QLD, Australia; [5]Division of Developmental Pediatrics, University of Virginia (UVA) School of Medicine and UVA Children's Hospital, Charlottesville, VA, USA

Clin Nutr 2013; 32: 579–584

Aims: The study aimed to evaluate: (1) the reliability of body impedance (BIA) measurements in young children with cerebral palsy (CP) across different grades of motor severity, (2) appropriate electrodes' placement for BIA in children with CP and unilateral involvement, (3) the best equation for the calculation of total body water (TBW) from the BIA in pre-school children with CP.

Methods: The study included 55 preschool children aged 2.40 ± 0.59 with CP and different ranges of Gross Motor Function Classification System (GMFCS) levels. Impedance (ohm) and TBW were measured and TBW was estimated from impedance using three previously published equations [19–21]. These equations were selected as they were all developed in groups containing children of preschool age and are all based on BIA.

Results: (1) Duplicate BIA measurements were performed in 50 children (91%) on the left-hand side of the body and 49 children on the right side. Duplicate measurements showed minimal differences: 0.5% variation on the left side of the body and 0.1% variation on the right side. However, there was a significant variation within some individuals and a third measurement was required in 44% measurements for the left-hand side and 35% occasions for the right-hand side of the body, since the duplicate measures were >5 ohm apart. (2) The mean differences of BIA results obtained from measurements conducted on either side of the body in young children with and without unilateral impairment were 1.2 and 0.8% respectively. (3) In children with bilateral impairment the estimated $\pm$ SD the mean of estimated and measures TBW $\pm$ SD were greatest for the Pencharz equations (10.4 ± 1.5 and 9.0 ± 1.4, respectively) and lowest for the Fjeld equation (7.6 ± 1.1 and

7.6 ± 1.2, respectively). In children with unilateral impairment, estimated TBW was lowest on the impaired compared to the unimpaired sides of the body for all three equations. Mean differences between the impaired and unimpaired sides were: for the Kushner equation: 0.3 liter (3%) (t = 2.55, p < 0.02); for the Pencharz equation: 0.5 liter (4%) (t = 4.53, p < 0.00), and for the Fjeld equation: 0.2 liter (2%) (t = 4.52, p < 0.00).

Conclusions: The ability of BIA to assess TBW accurately depended on the equation chosen. The Fjeld equation proved highly accurate at the population level for both children with bilateral and unilateral impairment, although individual results varied by up to 18%.

Micronutrient, antioxidant, and oxidative stress status in children with severe cerebral palsy

Schoendorfer NC[1], Vitetta L[2], Sharp N[1], DiGeronimo M[3], Wilson G[3], Coombes JS[3], Boyd R[4], Davies PS[1]

[1]Children's Nutrition Research Centre, The University of Queensland, Brisbane, QLD, Australia; [2]Centre for Integrative and Molecular Medicine, The University of Queensland, Brisbane, QLD, Australia; [3]Exercise and Oxidative Stress Research Group, School of Human Movements, The University of Queensland, Brisbane, QLD, Australia; [4]Queensland Cerebral Palsy and Rehabilitation Research Centre, The University of Queensland, Brisbane, QLD, Australia

JPEN J Parenter Enteral Nutr 2013; 37: 97–101

Aims: The study evaluated the micronutrient and antioxidant status in children with CP.

Methods: Red cell folate (RCF), magnesium, superoxide dismutase (SOD), glutathione reductase, and peroxidase, as well as serum methylmalonic acid and vitamin C were measured. Plasma hemoglobin, C-reactive protein, α-tocopherol, cholesterol, zinc, protein carbonyls, and total antioxidant capacity were also quantified in 24 children with CP and 24 typically developing healthy children, aged 4–12 years.

Results: There were no significant differences between the groups for concentrations of red cell glutathione peroxidase, red cell magnesium, hemoglobin z-score, serum α-tocopherol z-score/ cholesterol z-score ratio, protein carbonyl, or total antioxidant capacity. Red cell glutathione reductase (U/g Hb) was lower in orally-fed children compared with the other children (12.22 ± 2.41 in CP tube-fed vs. 10.15 ± 1.69 in CP orally-fed vs. 11.51 ± 1.67 in controls, p < 0.05). SOD activity (U/mg Hb) was also found significantly reduced in the enterally-fed children compared with the other groups (24.3 ± 1.4 in CP tube-fed vs. 25.7 ± 1.8 in CP orally-fed vs. 27.0 ± 2.8 in controls, p < 0.05). Plasma zinc z-score was found to be lower in the orally-fed group (−1.05 ± 0.73 in CP tube-fed vs. −1.10 ± 0.83 in CP orally-fed vs. −0.54 ± 0.54 in controls, p < 0.05). Red cell folate (nmol/l) was significantly higher in the enterally fed group (1,422 ± 70 in CP tube-fed vs. 843 ± 80 in CP orally-fed vs. 820 ± 43 in controls, p < 0.001), whereas MMA (nmol/l) was lower in this group, suggesting adequate B$_{12}$ status (88 ± 21 in CP tube-fed vs. 142 ± 101 in CP orally-fed vs. 157 ± 84 in controls, p < 0.05).

Conclusions: This study demonstrates a range of nutrition imbalances between tube-fed and orally-fed children with CP and TDC. Orally-fed children particularly showed several micronutrient deficiencies and enterally-fed children displayed certain excesses. Assessment of nutrient quality and not only quantity is obviously important in children with CP, either fed by tube or orally.

Fractures in children with cerebral palsy: a total population study

Uddenfeldt Wort U[1], Nordmark E[2], Wagner P[3], Düppe H[4], Westbom L[5]

[1]Department of Clinical Sciences, Social Medicine and Global Health, Lund University, Malmo, Sweden; [2]Department of Health Sciences, Health Sciences Centre, Lund University, Lund, Sweden; [3]National Centre for Quality Registers Skane University Hospital, Lund, Sweden; [4]Department of Orthopaedics Skane University Hospital, Malmo, Sweden; [5]Division of Paediatrics, Department of Clinical Sciences, Lund University, Lund, Sweden

Dev Med Child Neurol 2013; 55: 821–826

Aims: The study aimed to evaluate the prevalence, the type and the risk factors for fractures in children with CP compared to typically developed children (TDC).

Methods: The study is based on the data from the Skane CPUP programme, an epidemiological population study from Skane, Sweden, that collected data on body function, activity, and treatment in a CP follow-up registry. The present paper reported retrospective information on fracture events in children and young adults with CP born 1990–2005.

Results: The study population included 536 children (214 females): 11% were thin (BMI <-2 SD), 8% were obese (BMI >2 SD) and 12% were stunted. There were 103 fractures in 79 children, 13 children had more than one fracture. 19 (18%) occurred without any known trauma, 2 (2%) were in children in GMFCS levels I–III and 17 (16%) in children in GMFCS levels IV–V; 56 (54%) occurred after slight and 28 (27%) after moderate trauma. The majority of fractures occurred in children in GMFCS level I, and the fractures without trauma were most common in children with spastic CP and those in GMFCS levels IV–V. Of the 15 fractures of the femur, 14 occurred in children in GMFCS levels IV–V, and in 11 of those cases there was no known trauma involved. Children classified in GMFCS levels IV–V on antiepileptic drugs had a twofold increased ($p = 0.004$) fracture risk. The risk for fractures without trauma was also increased in stunted growth (height for age <-3SD) and for those who did not use standing devices, adjusted incidence ratio (AIRR) 4.16 ($p = 0.011$) and 3.66 ($p = 0.010$), respectively. The risk of fractures in gastrostomy-fed children was reduced for fractures with trauma, but increased for fractures without trauma (AIRR 0.10, $p = 0.003$ and 4.36, $p = 0.012$), respectively. The risk for fractures for children in GMFCS levels I–III was not significantly associated with any of the studied risk factors.

Conclusions: Children with CP with severe functional disabilities are at increased risk of fractures, especially if they are on antiepileptic drugs, stunted, do not use standing devices and are malnourished.

Timing of gastrostomy insertion in children with a neurodisability: a cross-sectional study of early versus late intervention

Sharma R[1], Williams AN[1], Zaw W[2]

[1]Department of Paediatrics, Virtual Academic Unit, Child Development Centre, Northampton, UK; [2]Department of Paediatrics, Northampton General Hospital, Northampton, UK

BMJ Open 2012; 2: e001793

Aims: The study aimed to evaluate whether early nutritional support using gastrostomy feeding in children with neurologic disabilities resulted in better weight gain and health outcome.

Methods: This was a retrospective, cross-sectional study which reviewed the pre- and post-gastrostomy weight and health outcome (hospitalization days) in 24 children who had gastrostomy placed before the age of 18 months and 17 children who had the gastrostomy placed after the age of 18 months.

Results: The mean weight pre-gastrostomy z-score in the <18 month group was −2.78 SD and −1.17 SD in the >18 month group. The mean weight post-gastrostomy z-score in the <18 month group was −1.45 SD and −0.72 SD in the >18 month group. The weight pre-gastrostomy z-score was significantly lower in the younger age group ($p = 0.014$), however there was no significant difference in z-score between the groups post-gastrostomy ($p = 0.178$). The mean difference in the z-score pre- and post-gastrostomy was significantly greater in the younger age group than in the older group ($p = 0.021$). There was no significant difference in the hospital admission rates pre- and post-gastrostomy in the early or the late group.

Conclusions: The results of the study shows that gastrostomy use for nutritional support improved weight gain at any age, but younger children achieved greater weight gain.

Gastrostomy tube feeding of children with cerebral palsy: variation across six European countries

Dahlseng MO[1], Andersen GL[2], Da Graca Andrada M[3], Arnaud C[4], Balu R[5], De la Cruz J[6], Folha T[7], Himmelmann K[8] Horridge K[9], Júlíusson PB[10], Påhlman M[8], Rackauskaite G[11], Sigurdardottir S[12], Uldall P[13], Vik T[1], Surveillance of Cerebral Palsy in Europe Network

[1]Department of Laboratory Medicine, Children's and Women's Health, Faculty of Medicine, Norwegian University of Science and Technology, Trondheim, Norway; [2]The Cerebral Palsy Registry of Norway, Vestfold Hospital Trust, Tønsberg, Norway; [3]The Cerebral Palsy Registry of Portugal, Federacao das Associacoes Portuguesas de Paralisia Cerebral, Lisbon, Portugal; [4]Inserm, UMR 1027, Toulouse, France; [5]Paediatric Department, Sunderland Royal Hospital, Sunderland, UK; [6]Clinical Research Unit, Imas12-Ciberesp, Hospital 12 Octubre, Madrid, Spain; [7]Calouste Gulbenkian Cerebral Palsy Rehabilitation Centre, Lisbon, Portugal; [8]Department of Pediatrics, Institute of Clinical Sciences, Queen Silvia Children's Hospital, Sahlgrenska Academy at the University of Gothenburg, Gothenburg, Sweden; [9]City Hospitals Sunderland NHS Foundation Trust, and North of England Collaborative Cerebral Palsy Survey, Sunderland, UK; [10]Department of Paediatrics, Haukeland University Hospital, Bergen, Norway; [11]Department of Paediatrics, Aarhus University Hospital, Aarhus, Denmark; [12]State Diagnostic, Counselling Centre, Kopavogur, Iceland; [13]Child Department, Righospitalet, Copenhagen University, Copenhagen, Denmark

Dev Med Child Neurol 2012; 54: 938–944

Aims: The aims of the study were to evaluate the approach to feeding difficulties and the indications for gastrostomy tube feeding (GTF) in children with CP in different European centers.

Methods: The study was part of the Surveillance of Cerebral Palsy in Europe Network (SCPE-NET), a 3-year programme based on the Surveillance of Cerebral Palsy in Europe, a collaboration of 21 registers in 13 European countries aimed at promoting best practice in the care of children with CP. Children with all CP subtypes and all GMFCS levels, born from 1999 to 2001, were included in the study. The primary outcome was the presence of a GTF. Secondary outcomes were age at placement of gastrostomy, growth and feeding difficulties.

Results: A total of 1,295 children (754 males, 541 females; mean age 5.11 years, range 6 months to 11.8 years) were included in this study. There were significant differences between areas in the proportions of various CP subtypes and GMFCS levels. In all, 133/1,295 (11%) children had a gastrostomy tube placed (22% in Sweden to 3% in Iceland). Gastrostomy feeding was given to 67% of children with GMFCS level IV and V in western Sweden, but only to 12% of children in Portugal. Median age at placement of gastrostomy was 22 months (range 1–120). The median age range between different countries was 16 months in western Sweden (5–108 months) to 70 months in northern England (12–120 months). The mean z-scores for weight was –0.86 (SD 1.71) and –0.87 for height (SD 1.50). In children in GMFCS level IV and V, there were significant differences in z-scores for weight and height between the areas. Portuguese children had lower weight z-scores compared with Norwegian, Swedish and Danish children ($p < 0.001$), while their height z-scores were lower only compared with Swedish and Danish children ($p = 0.002$). For children in GMFCS levels I and II, no significant differences in weight ($p = 0.114$) or height ($p = 0.472$) z-scores were observed between the different populations. The differences in z-scores between the countries were more marked when using the WHO growth references and also resulted in statistically significant differences for height z-scores between countries among children in GMFCS levels I and II.

Conclusions: The study showed considerable variations in the prevalence of growth restriction, feeding difficulties and the use of GTF in children with CP across different areas in six European countries. The differences were even more marked in children with GMFCS levels IV and V, the group most likely to have associated feeding difficulties. Among these children, those living in areas where GTF was less used were more growth-restricted than children in countries where GTF was more prevalent. This study outlines the lack of clear guidelines and differences in the decision-making with regard to nutritional support of children with CP in different centers.

Comments   Children with neurologic disabilities present complex management challenges, both for their families and for the professionals involved in their care. Growth retardation and feeding disorders are common in these children and represent a particular challenge to clinicians providing nutritional support. The first difficulty to face is to accurately assess the child's height and weight, which may not be possible using standard methods; therefore, proxies such as arm span or knee height may be required. The second challenge is to correctly assess their energy and nutrient needs to avoid over- or underprovision of nutrients. The single previous study that evaluated the EI in children with CP reported 44–54% overestimation compared to TEE data [18]. These differences could be explained by different populations or accuracy of food intake assessment and reporting. The significance of these discrepancies is that nutrition support should be based on objective and individualized evaluation in each child with CP, as generalizing data from different studies or populations may be subject to large deviations from the actual requirements.

Historical cohorts demonstrate significant levels of malnutrition, however the clinician has to be aware that some children may not follow a standard growth trajectory and follow a growth trajectory set by their own genetic potential/disease. Several studies have shown that body composition and resting energy expenditure (REE) is variable in children with cerebral palsy (CP) and are affected by multiple factors (functional capacity, degree of mobility, severity of disease, level of altered metabolism disease, medication, type of feeding, etc.). Height and weight are not necessarily reliable predictors of REE with most studies demonstrating significantly lower REE than expected or compared with control groups. Total energy expenditure (TEE) is generally (although not always) reduced in children with neurologic disability; those with the most severe motor impairment having the lowest TEE. As illustrated by the study of Walker et al., direct measurement of REE in children with CP is therefore the only reliable way to accurately evaluate energy needs. Measurement of body composition is an indispensable component of nutritional assessment and is paramount to the success of any nutritional program. There are few studies incorporating body composition analysis in assessment of the nutritional status of children with CP. The study of Bell et al. reported the calculated values of body water spaces (from BIA) and compared them with the measured values (from dilution isotopes) and good concordance (differences against mean) was reported, suggesting that BIA is a reliable method for estimating total body water and extracellular water in children with CP.

Evaluation of bone mineral density is another important aspect of nutrition evaluation of children with neurologic disabilities. The study of Uddenfeldt Wort et al. reports on the risk factors associated with fractures in a population of children with CP and different degrees of functional disabilities. The availability of new techniques, such peripheral quantitative CT, will improve our ability to diagnose poor bone quality and timely identify the children at risk of fractures.

The other studies presented in this chapter demonstrate furthermore the contradictions among the health caregivers with regard to nutritional support (type and timing) of children with CP. Lack of an objective measure of nutritional needs and clear guidelines of when and how and what to give for nutritional support are evident obstacles for appropriate care.

Future studies should address the particularities of energy metabolism and its regulation in this population. When adequately nourished, children and adolescents with cerebral palsy appear more tranquil and require decreased feeding time, which gives caregivers time to develop the child's functional independence and character. Understanding energy requirements of this population will provide caregivers and health professionals with guidelines for providing and promoting optimal nutritional status.

Autistic Spectrum Disorders

Early Growth Patterns in Children with Autism

Surén P[1,2], Stoltenberg C[2], Bresnahan M[3,4], Hirtz D[5], Lie KK[2], Lipkin WI[3], Magnus P[2], Reichborn-Kjennerud T[2,6], Schjølberg S[2], Susser E[3,4], Oyen AS[2,7], Li L[1], Hornig M[3]

[1]Centre for Paediatric Epidemiology and Biostatistics, UCL Institute of Child Health, London, UK; [2]The Norwegian Institute of Public Health, Oslo, Norway; [3]The Mailman School of Public Health, Columbia University, New York, NY, USA; [4]New York State Psychiatric Institute, New York, NY, USA; [5]National Institute of Neurological Disorders and Stroke, Bethesda, MD, USA; [6]Institute of Psychiatry, University of Oslo, Oslo, Norway; [7]Nic Waals Institute, Lovisenberg Hospital, Oslo, Norway

Epidemiology 2013; 24: 660–670

Aims: The study reports the data from the population-based longitudinal Norwegian Mother and Child Cohort Study (MoBa) on growth pattern of head circumference (HC), length, and weight in children with autism spectrum disorders (ASD).

Methods: The MoBa cohort is a Norwegian nationwide registry and includes 109,000 children born from 1999 to 2009. Cases of ASD in the cohort were identified by a substudy of autism, the Autism

Birth Cohort Study. Growth trajectories were modeled using mixed-effects models to take into account the within-subject correlation of head and body sizes.

Results: A total of 376 children in the study sample (106,082 children) had been diagnosed with ASD (310 boys and 66 girls). The mean birth HC in boys was not different in children with or without ADS. The mean HC in boys was similar after birth in cases and non-cases (HC mean difference <0.1 cm), but the variability of HC was greater in cases and there was an increase in the proportion with macrocephaly in ASD boys by age 12 months, to 8.7% (4.7–14.4%). The difference between cases and non-cases in girls reached 0.5 cm at 12 months of age. Adjustment for covariates attenuated the difference to 0.2 cm at 12 months. Boys with ASD had similar lengths to non-cases at birth, but grew faster after birth and were taller by 0.5 cm at 6 months and 1.1 cm at 12 months, but the mean difference reverted to 0.6 cm by age 3 years. In girls with ASD the mean birth length was 0.64 cm lower than the mean for girls without ASD but the differences in means were smaller at other ages. The birth weight of boys with ASD was similar to birth weight in non-cases, but after birth, ASD boys had a more rapid increase in mean weight and were on average about 300 g heavier than other boys from age 12 months. In girls with ASD, mean birth weight was lower than the mean for other girls and continued to be 150–350 g lower up to age 3 years, but the difference in means largely disappeared after adjustment for covariates. Boys with ASD had similar mean BMIs to other boys at all ages. Girls with ASD had somewhat lower mean BMIs throughout, as a result of their lower mean weight, although the 95% CIs were always overlapping with those of non-cases.

Conclusions: Growth trajectories for HC, length and weight in children with ASD were different from those of other children and the differences are sex-specific. Boys showed higher prevalence of macrocephaly and increased mean length and weight up to 12 months. For girls with ASD, the reductions in length, weight, and HC were attenuated by adjustment for covariates.

Nutrition, physical activity, and bone mineral density in youth with autistic spectrum disorders

Soden SE[1], Garrison CB[1], Egan AM[1], Beckwith AM[2]

[1]Section of Developmental and Behavioral Sciences, Department of Pediatrics, Children's Mercy Hospitals and Clinics, Kansas City, MO, USA; [2]Department of Neurodevelopmental Pediatrics, Children's Specialized Hospital, Mountainside, Mountainside, NJ, USA

J Dev Behav Pediatr 2012; 33: 618–624

Aims: The aim of the study was to (1) assess the nutritional intake of children with ASDs, (2) evaluate bone mineral density (BMD) in a sample of 10- to 18-year-olds with ASDs, and (3) correlate medical history and body mass index (BMI), diet, activity, and parental perceptions of lifestyle with BMD.

Methods: The study included 26 children aged 10–18 years with ASDs. Anthropometries, Tanner stage, medication and medical diagnoses ware collected by parent interview and from the clinic record. Parents were asked to rate their child's dietary habits, their average physical activity level and to estimate the sunlight exposure in a typical week. Dual-energy x-ray absorptiometery (DXA) was used to measure BMD of the lumbar spine (L1–L4). Laboratory tests included serum 25-OHD, alkaline phosphatase, parathyroid hormone, erythrocyte indices, electrolytes, liver and renal function tests, thyroid-stimulating hormone, and free T_4.

Results: There were 21 males (80.8%) and 5 females (19.2%) aged from 10.3 to 18.2 years (mean 13.4). Mean body mass index (BMI) percentile was 47.9 (SD 36.37, range 1st to 99th), 27% of participants were overweight, while 23% were underweight. Food diaries indicated that participants'

intakes were deficient for several nutrients including vitamins A, B_3, D, E, K, zinc, calcium, folate, fiber and potassium. The mean BMD z-score was –0.1 (SD 1.51, range –3.3 to –2.7). Four participants (15%) had a z-score ≤ -2.0. BMD was significantly positively correlated with BMI percentile (r = 0.47, p < 0.05), percent of recommended calcium intake (r = 0.46, p < 0.05), and percent of recommended caloric intake (r = 0.58, p < 0.01) calculated from diet diaries.

Conclusions: Children and adolescents with ASDs are at risk of low BMD due to their low calcium and vitamin D intake. Screening for low BMD should be therefore performed in children with ASDs based on an understanding of which patients are at greatest risk.

Nutrient intake from food in children with autism

Hyman SL[1], Stewart PA[1,2], Schmidt B[1], Cain U[3], Lemcke N[1], Foley JT[1], Peck R[2], Clemons T[4], Reynolds A[5], Johnson C[6,7], Handen B[7], James SJ[8], Courtney PM[9], Molloy C[1], Ng PK[1]

[1]Department of Pediatrics, University of Rochester Medical Center, Rochester, NY, USA; [2]Clinical and Translational Science Institute, University of Rochester School of Medicine, Rochester, NY, USA; [3]Boston University School of Medicine, Boston, MA, USA; [4]EMMES Corporation, Baltimore, MD, USA; [5]Department of Pediatrics, University of Colorado School of Medicine, Denver, CO, USA; [6]Department of Pediatrics, University of Pittsburgh School of Medicine, Pittsburgh, PA, USA; [7]Department of Psychiatry, University of Pittsburgh School of Medicine, Pittsburgh, PA, USA; [8]Department of Pediatrics, University of Arkansas for Medical Sciences, Little Rock, AR, USA; [9]Department of Pediatrics, University of Cincinnati College of Medicine, Cincinnati, OH, USA

Pediatrics 2012; 130(suppl 2): S145–S153

Aims: The study evaluated the food intake of children with autism spectrum disorders (ASD) and compared it to food intake the general pediatric population by using the National Health and Nutrition Examination Survey (NHANES) data.

Methods: The study population was recruited among children treated at five Autism Treatment Network (ATN) sites. Height and weight were measured and BMI and BMI percentile were calculated. Parents completed a 3-day food record containing all foods, beverages and supplements ingested by the child over 3 consecutive days.

Results: The study enrolled 367 children with ASD (2–11 years); nutrition data were based on 252 food records. Dietary restriction of gluten, casein, or processed sugars was reported by 18% of participants. Use of food supplement (vitamins, minerals, herbal, or botanical compounds) was reported by 66% of study participants, compared with 35% in the NHANES and 61% in a national sample of children with chronic disease. Compared to children in NHANES, children with ASDs aged 2–5 years were more likely to be overweight (p < 0.05) or obese (p < 0.001) and children aged 6–11 years were proportionately more underweight (p < 0.05). Children on restricted diets were more likely to be underweight than those not on restricted diets (p = 0.02). Macronutrient intakes were within the acceptable macronutrient distribution range by age, however children with ASDs (ages 4–8 years) consumed less energy, lower percentage of protein and greater percentage of carbohydrates than the NHANES (2007–2008) matched sample. Children with ASDs had lower intakes of vitamin D (2–11 years), lower levels of phosphorus intake (9–11 years) and reported lower intakes of vitamin A, vitamin C, and zinc compared with the NHANES controls. Many children with ASDs have intakes above the upper limit, from food alone, for micronutrients such as copper, retinol (vitamin A), folic acid, zinc, and manganese.

Conclusions: The data from this study shows that overweight and underweight, as well as micronutrient deficiencies or excesses are prevalent among children with ASDs. These results indicate the importance of nutritional surveillance in primary care for all children, especially children with ASDs. The best way to achieve that is periodic dietary assessment corroborated with anthropometric and laboratory data, and consideration of referral to a registered dietitian.

Iron status in children with autism spectrum disorder

Reynolds A[1], Krebs NF[1], Stewart PA[2], Austin H[1], Johnson SL[1], Withrow N[1], Molloy C[3], James SJ[4], Johnson C[5], Clemons T[6], Schmidt B[2], Hyman SL[2]

[1]Department of Pediatrics, University of Colorado, Denver, CO, USA; [2]Department of Pediatrics, University of Rochester, Rochester, NY, USA; [3]Department of Pediatrics, Cincinnati Children's Hospital Medical Center, Cincinnati, OH, USA; [4]Department of Pediatrics, University of Arkansas, Little Rock, AR, USA; [5]Department of Pediatrics, University of Pittsburgh, Pittsburgh, PA, USA; [6]EMMES Corporation, Rockville, MD, USA

Pediatrics 2012; 130(suppl 2): S154–S159

Aims: The study aims were to determine the prevalence of iron deficiency in children with ASD and evaluate the iron intake, and the relationship of iron intake to iron status.

Methods: The study population was recruited among children treated at five Autism Treatment Network (ATN) sites. Parents completed a 3-day food record containing all foods, beverages, and supplements ingested by the child over 3 consecutive days. Laboratory tests included complete blood count, serum ferritin (SF), transferring saturation (TS), iron, and total iron-binding capacity (TIBC).

Results: Iron status was evaluated in 222/368 (60%, mean age 5.3 years, range 2–11) children with ASDs enrolled in the Diet and Nutrition Study. Low iron stores were found in 8% of children (SF <12 ng/ml). One child had IDA. ID rates were lower in all age groups of children with ASDs, compared with NHANES data. The percentage of children with iron intakes less than EAR was 2% and increased with age. Children with ASD did not differ from the NHANES population in iron intake. The major sources of iron in the diet of these children were from enriched or fortified foods, such as breakfast cereals.

Conclusions: Children with ASD have low iron intakes and are at risk for low SF. Taking into consideration the important consequences of iron deficiency on developmental and behavioral function in infants and children, dietary history and screening for iron stores should be considered in children with ASD and inadequate iron intake.

Comments   Autism spectrum disorders (ASD) are neurodevelopmental disorders characterized by impaired social and communication interactions as well as limited, repetitive interests and behavior. The longitudinal population-based Norwegian registry reported that children with ASD also have different growth trajectories when compared to other children.

Conventional treatment is based on the combination of behavioral and pharmacotherapy. Dietary manipulations are frequently adopted by families of children with ASD seeking to improve their children behavior. Dietary manipulations in conjunction with children's peculiar feeding habits may easily result in multiple nutritional deficiencies, undernutrition or overweight and poor bone status, as illustrated by the studies published this last year. An important part of autism children's care is evaluation and support of patient's nutritional status to prevent further neurological and behavior deterioration as a result of nutritional deficiencies. Many studies have shown the need to supplement the missing nutrients from the diets of autistic patients with fatty acids omega-3, probiotics, vitamins and minerals. Adopted diets should take into consideration nutritional requirements and food preferences of the patient. It is important to emphasize that continual monitoring of the diet and nutritional status of children with ASD is required. Parents and caregivers should be aware of the benefits and dangers of nutritional manipulations and the need for proper monitoring of diet and growth of children with ASD.

Anorexia Nervosa

Growth hormone level at admission and its evolution during refeeding are predictive of short-term outcome in restrictive anorexia nervosa

Nogueira JP[1], Valéro R[1,2], Maraninchi M[1], Lorec AM[3], Samuelian-Massat C[2], Bégu-Le Corroller A[2], Nicolay A[1,3], Gaudart J[4], Portugal H[1,3], Vialettes B[1,2]

[1]UMR 1062 INSERM/1260 INRA, Aix-Marseille University, Marseille, France; [2]Department of Nutrition, Metabolic Diseases and Endocrinology, APHM, La Timone Hospital, Aix-Marseille University, Marseille, France; [3]Department of Biochemistry, APHM, La Timone Hospital, Aix-Marseille University, Marseille, France; [4]Biostatistics Research Unit (LERTIM), Faculty of Medicine, APHM, Aix-Marseille University, Marseille, France

Br J Nutr 2013; 109: 2175–2181

Aims: Investigation of prognostic value of GH, IGF-1 levels, adipocytokine profiles, insulin sensitivity, body composition and energy expenditure on the outcome in restrictive anorexia nervosa (AN).

Methods: Eleven patients diagnosed with AN (age 21 ± 0.39 years) and 10 healthy age-matched young women aged were studied at admission (T0, BMI 16), at discharge, (T2, BMI 17.5) and at 6 months after discharge (T3).

Results: At baseline (T0), plasma GH and serum ghrelin levels were higher in AN patients compared with controls ($p < 0.05$ for both). Plasma levels of IGF-1, estradiol, free tri-iodothyronine (fT_3), leptin and adiponectin were significantly lower in patients with AN compared with control subjects ($p < 0.05$ for all). Plasma levels of glucose, insulin and HOMA-IR were also significantly lower in patients with AN than in control subjects ($p < 0.05$ for all). At the first stage of refeeding (T1) body fat mass (BFM) and body lean mass, resting energy expenditure (REE), active energy expenditure and total energy expenditure (TEE) increased significantly ($p < 0.05$ for all). A significant decrease in GH, ghrelin and testosterone levels and an increase in IGF-1 fT_3 and estradiol concentrations were observed ($p < 0.05$ for all). A significant increase was only seen with adiponectin ($p < 0.05$). There was a significant increase in glucose, insulin and HOMA-IR levels ($p < 0.05$ for all). At T1, there was a significant negative association between GH and plasma glucose levels and between GH levels and active energy expenditure ($r = 0.7$, $p < 0.04$ and $r = 0.8$, $p < 0.02$, respectively). At T2 stage of refeeding (T1) REE increased significantly ($p < 0.05$). There was a significant increase in IGF-1 and leptin levels ($p < 0.05$ for both). Glucose and HOMA-IR levels increased significantly ($p < 0.05$ for both). Plasma GH levels were negatively and significantly associated with leptin levels ($r = 0.8$, $p < 0.03$). At 6 months after discharge with a BMI >17.5 ($\Delta = T2-T0$), stepwise multivariate analysis showed that GH was the strongest determinant of BMI at T3, accounting for 74% of its variability ($r = 0.74$, $p < 0.05$).

Conclusions: GH level at admission was an important contributor in the variability of the final BMI. GH at admission and evolution during refeeding may predict short-term clinical outcome after weight recuperation. Specifically, low GH levels at admission in hospital and lower amplitude of plasma GH variation between admission and discharge from hospital were strongly associated with relapse 6 months after discharge.

Linear growth and final height characteristics in adolescent females with anorexia nervosa

Modan-Moses D[1,3], Yaroslavsky A[2], Kochavi B[2], Toledano A[2], Segev S[2], Balawi F[2], Mitrany E[2], Stein D[2,3]

[1]Pediatric Endocrinology and Diabetes Unit, The Edmond and Lily Safra Children's Hospital, The Chaim Sheba Medical Center, Tel-Hashomer, Ramat Gan, Israel; [2]Pediatric Psychosomatic Department, The Edmond and Lily Safra Children's Hospital, The Chaim Sheba Medical Center, Tel-Hashomer, Ramat Gan, Israel; [3]The Sackler School of Medicine, Tel Aviv University, Tel Aviv, Israel

PLoS One 2012; 7: e45504

Aim: The aim of this study was to assess linear growth and final height in female adolescent inpatients with anorexia nervosa (AN).

Methods: This retrospective study reviewed all the medical charts of female patients hospitalized for the treatment of AN between 1/1/1987 and 31/12/1999. Pre-morbid and admission height and weight measurements were obtained from patients' files. Final height (defined as height at age 18 or older, and at least 3 years after menarche) was measured in 69 patients 2–10 years following discharge from their index hospitalization.

Results: The mean age of the 211 patients on admission was 16.6 ± 4.2 years; the mean BMI was 15.7 ± 1.02, and the mean age at menarche was 12.7 ± 2.4 years. The mean height SDS on admission was -0.285 ± 1.02, and increased during hospitalization to -0.271 ± 1.02. Final height was available for 69 patients (32.7%). On admission, the mean height SDS of these 69 patients was -0.231 ± 1.103. During hospitalization, height SDS increased to -0.197 ± 1.122. Mean final height SDS was -0.258 ± 1.04 (161.6 ± 6.8 cm), which, similar to the admission and discharge height SDS, was significantly lower than expected in a normal population ($p = 0.04$). Height SDS on admission was a strong predictor of final height SDS ($p < 0.001$). A significant ($p = 0.019$) interaction was found between final height and pubertal status at admission. Patients admitted less than 1 year after menarche showed less catch-up growth and their final height was more severely compromised in comparison to patients admitted more than 1 year after menarche.

Conclusions: Growth retardation is present female adolescents with AN and affects final height, especially of younger adolescents. It seems that in order to achieve height catch-up to the pre-morbid percentile pre-morbid growth data should be obtained, and target weight should be based on the expected, rather than the measured height percentile at the time of diagnosis.

Comments Anorexia nervosa (AN) is a psychiatric disorder that occurs mainly in female adolescents and young women. The obsessive fear of weight gain, critically limited food intake and neuroendocrine aberrations characteristic of AN have both short- and long-term consequences for the reproductive, cardiovascular, gastrointestinal and skeletal systems. The short-term, life-threatening complications include electrolyte abnormalities and cardiac complications such as sinus bradycardia, a prolonged QT interval on electrocardiography, arrhythmias, myocardial mass modification and hypotension.

Decrease in bone mineral density and the increased risk of spontaneous fractures are some of the most important medical consequences of AN. To this we should add growth retardation and lower final adult height, as shown by the study by of Modan-Moses et al. The treatment of AN should therefore aim not only at fast recovery but also to prevent and treat the long-term effects of this disorder. Monitoring GH levels at admission and during refeeding in patients suffering from AN was shown to have some prognostic value. The role of this factor in the disease is however, probably indirect, reflecting specific changes associated with the adapted response to starvation. Further investigations of the long-term disease risk of relapse and the approach to their prevention and treatment are needed.

References

1 Pfefferkorn M, Burke G, Griffiths A, Markowitz J, Rosh J, Mack D, et al: Growth abnormalities persist in newly diagnosed children with Crohn disease despite current treatment paradigms. J Pediatr Gastroenterol Nutr 2009;48:168–174.

2 Sawczenko A, Ballinger AB, Savage MO, Sanderson IR: Clinical features affecting final adult height in patients with pediatric-onset Crohn's disease. Pediatr 2006;118:124–129.

3 Hanning RM, Blimkie CJR, Bar-Or O, Lands LC, Moss LA, Wilson WM: Relationships among nutritional status and skeletal and respiratory muscle function in cystic fibrosis: does early dietary supplementation make a difference? Am J Clin Nutr 1993; 57:580–587.

4 Kalnins D, Corey M, Ellis L, Pencharz PB, Tullis E, Durie PR: Failure of conventional strategies to improve nutritional status in malnourished adolescents and adults with cystic fibrosis. J Pediatr 2005;147: 399–401.

5 Poustie VJ, Russell JE, Watling RM, Ashby D, Smyth RL, on behalf of the CALICO Trial Collaborative Group: Oral protein energy supplements for children with cystic fibrosis: CALICO multicentre randomised controlled trial. BMJ 2006;332:632–636.

6 Schnabel D, Grasemann C, Staab D, Wollmann H, Ratjen F: A multicenter, randomized, double-blind, placebo-controlled trial to evaluate the metabolic and respiratory effects of growth hormone in children with cystic fibrosis. Pediatrics 2007;119:e1230–e1238.

7 Stalvey MS, Anbar RD, Konstan MW, Jacobs JR, Bakker B, Lippe B, Geller DE: A multi-center controlled trial of growth hormone treatment in children with cystic fibrosis. Pediatr Pulmonol 2012;47: 252–263.

8 Hütler M, Schnabel D, Staab D, Tacke A, Wahn U, Boning D, Beneke R: Effect of growth hormone on exercise tolerance in children with cystic fibrosis. Med Sci Sports Exerc 2002;34:567–572.

9 Schibler A, von der Heiden R, Birrer P, Mullis PE: Prospective randomised treatment with recombinant human growth hormone in cystic fibrosis. Arch Dis Child 2003;88:1078–1081.

10 Corey M, McLaughlin FJ, Williams M, Levison H: A comparison of survival, growth, and pulmonary function in patients with cystic fibrosis in Boston and Toronto. J Clin Epidemiol 1988;41:583–591.

11 Stallings VA, Stark LJ, Robinson KA, Feranchak AP, Quinton H: Evidence-based practice recommendations for nutrition-related management of children and adults with cystic fibrosis and pancreatic insufficiency: results of a systematic review. J Am Diet Assoc 2008;108:832–839.

12 Phung OJ, Coleman CI, Baker EL, Scholle JM, Girotto JE, Makanji SS, Chen WT, Talati R, Kluger J, White CM: Recombinant human growth hormone in the treatment of patients with cystic fibrosis. Pediatrics 2010;126:e1211–e1226.

13 Gaskin KJ: Nutritional care in children with cystic fibrosis: are our patients becoming better? Eur J Clin Nutr 2013;67:558–564.

14 Weir JBDV: New methods for calculating metabolic rate with special reference to protein metabolism. J Physiol 1949;109:1–9.

15 Rieken R, van Goudoever JB, Schierbeek H, Willemsen SP, Calis EAC, Tibboel D, Evenhuis HM, Penning C: Measuring body composition and energy expenditure in children with severe neurological impairment and intellectual disability. Am J Clin Nutr 2011;94:759–766.

16 Palisano R, Rosenbaum P, Walter S, Russell D, Wood E, Galuppi B: Development and reliability of a system to classify gross motor function in children with cerebral palsy. Dev Med Child Neurol 1997;39: 214–223.

17 Calis EAC, Veugelers R, Sheppard JJ, Tibboel D, Evenhuis HM, Penning C: Dysphagia in children with severe generalized cerebral palsy and intellectual disability. Dev Med Child Neurol 2008;50:625–630.

18 Stallings VA, Zemel BS, Davies JC, Cronk CE, Charney EB: Energy expenditure of children and adolescents with severe disabilities: a cerebral palsy model. Am J Clin Nutr 1996;64:627–634.

19 Kushner RF, Schoeller DA: Estimation of total body water by bioelectrical impedance analysis. Am J Clin Nutr 1986;44:417–424.

20 Pencharz PB, Azcue M: Use of bioelectrical impedance analysis measurements in the clinical management of malnutrition. Am J Clin Nutr 1996;64:485S–488S.

21 Fjeld C, Freundt-Thurne J, Schoeller D: Total body water measurement by [18]O dilution and bioelectrical impedance in well and malnourished children. Pediatr Res 1990;27:98–102.

Hartman/Altowati/Ahmed/Shamir

Koletzko B, Shamir R, Turck D, Phillip M (eds): Nutrition and Growth: Yearbook 2014.
World Rev Nutr Diet. Basel, Karger, 2014, vol 109, pp 89–100 (DOI: 10.1159/000356109)

Malnutrition and Catch-Up Growth during Childhood and Puberty

Youn Hee Jee[1], Jeffrey Baron[1], Moshe Phillip[2] and Zulfiqar A. Bhutta[3]

[1] National Institute of Child Health and Human Development, National Institutes of Health, Bethesda, MD, USA
[2] Jesse Z and Sara Lea Shafer Institute for Endocrinology and Diabetes, National Center for Childhood Diabetes, Schneider Children's Medical Center of Israel, Petach-Tikva and Sackler Faculty of Medicine, Tel Aviv University, Tel Aviv, Israel
[3] Robert Harding Chair in Global Child Health & Policy, Sick Kids Center for Global Child Health, Toronto, ON, Canada and Center of Excellence in Women and Child Health, The Aga Khan University, Karachi, Pakistan

This chapter reviews important recent papers related to catch-up growth. Catch-up growth is generally defined as body growth that (1) is more rapid than normal for age and (2) follows a period of growth inhibition. As can be seen by the studies reviewed in this chapter, catch-up growth can occur after either pre- or postnatal growth inhibition, can show a variety of temporal patterns, and can be either complete (yielding a normal adult body size) or incomplete. These studies explore the implications of catch-up growth not only for adult body size but also for pubertal timing, bone strength, and the risk of metabolic syndrome.

Patterns of catch-up growth

De Wit CC[1], Sas TCJ[2,3], Wit JM[4], Cutfield WS[1]

[1] The Liggins Institute, University of Auckland, Auckland, New Zealand; [2] Department of Pediatrics, Albert Schweitzer Hospital, Dordrecht, The Netherlands; [3] Department of Pediatrics, Erasmus Medical Centre, Rotterdam, The Netherlands; [4] Department of Pediatrics, Leiden University Medical Center, Leiden, The Netherlands

J Pediatr 2013; 162: 415–420

Summary: This paper reviews the possible mechanisms, the precipitating conditions, and especially the temporal patterns of catch-up growth in children. There are two principal hypotheses to explain catch-up growth – central nervous system sensing of expected body size and intrinsic capacity of the growth plate. Two temporal patterns of catch-up growth that were introduced by Tanner were discussed. The type A pattern is a transient increase in growth velocity after cessation of the growth restriction, followed by normal growth velocity when the original growth curve is achieved. The type B pattern shows a slightly greater growth velocity than expected for chronological age but a normal growth velocity for bone age. This review article shows evidence that type A catch-up growth is seen in some children with hypothyroidism and with growth hormone deficiency, especially on higher doses of growth hormone. Type B catch-up growth has been demonstrated in a prospective study of celiac disease. The authors also propose an intermediate pattern of catch-up growth, which they term, 'type AB' which shows an increased growth velocity initially, followed by a stabilization of height SDS for years, and a delayed pubertal growth spurt, which brings the individual closer to target height. The authors indicate that this pattern is seen in some children with celiac disease, hypothyroidism, GH deficiency, and children born prematurely.

Comments   This review is a valuable synthesis of experience and data regarding catch-up growth, derived from a wide variety of sources. The proposed intermediate type AB catch-up growth pattern seems quite reasonable. Indeed it would be surprising if some children showed a type A pattern, some a type B pattern, but none showed an intermediate pattern. Unfortunately, as the authors observe, there are not much data that were collected systematically to rigorously define temporal patterns. Such data would have to include bone ages to distinguish whether a child's initial growth rate was greater than expected for bone age indicating a type AB, rather than a type B pattern. Instead, we have mostly anecdotal reports and subjective impressions from looking at growth charts. The authors did analyze previously published data from children with treated growth hormone deficiency, which showed a mixture of type A and type AB patterns, with the A pattern occurring uniformly with higher doses. Unfortunately, growth hormone treatment of growth hormone deficiency is not the ideal model to study physiology because, as the authors point out, treatment does not necessarily restore physiological hormonal levels and therefore the pattern may be dependent on the dose chosen.

The temporal pattern of catch-up growth has interesting implications regarding the underlying mechanism. The type B pattern is consistent with the delayed growth plate senescence hypothesis which states that children undergo catch-up growth because the growth-inhibiting conditions have delayed the normal decline in growth plate function (which is approximately reflected by a delayed bone age). The type A pattern suggests that some other mechanism is at work. The type AB pattern might be explained by delayed growth plate senescence plus an additional mechanism.

The review is generally very thorough. However, it states that there are no reports on catch-up growth after discontinuation of exogenous glucocorticoid administration, whereas there are some data to be considered. For example, a systematic study of catch-up growth in 56 children with nephrotic syndrome [1] showed that catch-up growth occurred after withdrawal of prednisone treatment, although the catch-up growth appeared incomplete after 5 years of follow-up.

Catch-up in bone acquisition in young adult men with late normal puberty

Darelid A, Ohlsson C, Nilsson M, Kindblom JM, Mellström D, Lorentzon M

Centre for Bone and Arthritis Research, Institute of Medicine, Sahlgrenska University Hospital, Gothenburg, Sweden

J Bone Miner Res 2012; 27: 2198–2207

Background: Sex steroids at the time of puberty have a positive effect on bone density. In females, late menarche has been associated with lower BMD persisting into adulthood. The long-term effects of pubertal timing on the skeleton of young men has not been well established.

Methods: Subjects were from a population-based cohort from the Gothenburg Osteoporosis and Obesity Study. Areal bone mineral density (aBMD), bone mineral content (BMC), volumetric bone mineral density (vBMD) and cortical bone size were measured in 501 men between 19 and 24 years using dual-energy x-ray absorptiometry (DXA) and peripheral quantitative CT scan (pQCT) at baseline and at follow-up. Detailed growth and weight charts were used to calculate age at peak height velocity (PHV).

Results: Subjects were divided into three groups, those with early, middle and late puberty, according to age at PHV. There were no significant differences in age, calcium intake, or smoking between the groups. Age at PHV was a strong positive predictor of gain in bone mass. Thus, the group with late puberty gained markedly more in aBMD and BMC at the total body, radius, and lumbar spine, and lost less at the femoral neck than the group with early puberty. Age at PHV was also an independent positive predictor of the increase in cortical thickness and periosteal circumference of the radius, measured by pQCT. At age 24 years, no significant differences in aBMD or BMC of the lumbar spine, femoral neck, or total body were observed. pQCT measurements of the radius at follow-up also demonstrated no significant differences in bone size although cortical and trabecular vBMD were lower in men with late versus early puberty. Age at PHV was not associated with distal forearm fracture prevalence.

Conclusion: Late puberty in males was associated with a substantial catch-up in bone density and in bone thickness by young adulthood, leaving little or no deficits in the parameters studied.

Comments   The effects of pubertal timing on adult bone density are difficult to ascertain in human studies. In women, late puberty is associated with lower bone density persisting into adulthood. However, this association may not represent a cause-and-effect relationship between pubertal timing and adult BMD because the difference in BMD actually precedes the onset of puberty, suggesting that the later puberty and the persistent low BMD may both reflect genetic/nutritional/body mass effects [2]. In males, it is not clear whether pubertal timing is associated with persistent differences in BMD, or, if there is an association, whether there is a direct causal relationship.

In the study reviewed here, delayed puberty was associated with catch-up in aBMD, BMC and vBMD. One could argue that these increases in bone density should not be considered catch-up *growth*. Trabecular bone formation is a process that is not restricted to childhood but rather persists into adulthood, setting it apart from growth of many other structures. However, increasing bone width, which involves periosteal bone formation, is part of childhood growth, occurring rapidly during early years and slowing as adulthood approaches. One interesting finding from this study is that catch-up in the periosteal circumference of the radius also occurred. Thus, this study demonstrates that, in children with late puberty, catch-up growth occurs not only in linear bone growth (which determines height) but also in cross-sectional bone growth (which affects bone strength). Whether catch-up in bone width requires subsequent androgen exposure (which stimulates periosteal bone formation) is not known. Similarly, the mechanism of catch-up growth in bone width is unknown.

This study also argues against the widely stated notion that there is a 'golden window of opportunity' to lay down bone during adolescence. Contrary to this notion, when exposure to sex steroids occurs on the later side of the normal range, catch-up occurs, ultimately resulting in a skeleton that is normal, or nearly so.

Is early puberty triggered by catch-up growth following undernutrition?

Proos L, Gustafsson J

Department of Women's and Children's Health, Uppsala University, Uppsala, Sweden

Int J Environ Res Public Health 2012; 9: 1791–1809

Summary: This paper reviews catch-up growth after undernutrition and the relationship between catch-up growth and early pubertal development. Catch-up growth can occur following intrauterine growth restriction or after postnatal undernutrition (e.g. Crohn's disease, celiac disease or eating disorders) as well as after combined fetal-postnatal undernutrition when the subsequent nutritional intake is adequate. Catch-up growth may be associated with earlier timing of puberty after intrauterine growth retardation and after combined fetal-postnatal undernutrition. The authors state that catch-up growth following undernutrition that occurs only postnatally has not been reported to be associated with earlier pubertal development. Catch-up growth occurs when children are adopted from developing countries to developed countries and is associated with earlier puberty than that of the reference population. The mechanisms responsible for the association between catch-up growth and early puberty remain unknown. For international adoption, the hypotheses include both shifts in nutritional status and also endocrine-disrupting chemicals from pesticides.

Comments This review provides a valuable synthesis of studies linking catch-up growth and early puberty. One particularly interesting conclusion of this review is that early puberty has been observed after prenatal growth restriction or after combined pre- and postnatal restriction, but not after isolated postnatal undernutrition. Of course, lack of supporting evidence is not the same as evidence to the contrary. We do not have good studies of pubertal timing after transient postnatal growth restriction. In fact, even finding the right model to study a possible association is not easy. Most disorders that cause postnatal nutritional problems, such as gastrointestinal disease, may not resolve completely. International adoption can allow a recovery from postnatal undernutrition and is associated with early puberty in girls. Although exposure to endocrine-disrupting pesticides has been suggested as a possible etiology, the review mentions that, in one study, the girls with the most pronounced stunting and fastest catch-up growth had the lowest age of menarche, implicating the growth restriction in the etiology. The review points out that many international adoptees also had a low birth weight and thus were subject to combined fetal-postnatal undernutrition. However, not mentioned in the review is a study of 276 internationally adopted girls where those with a birth weight <2,500 g and those with a birth weight >2,500 g showed similar early pubertal development [3]. In our opinion, these data suggest, but do not prove, that early pubertal development is associated not only with catch-up growth after prenatal growth restriction but also after postnatal undernutrition.

Revisiting the relationship of weight and height in early childhood

Richard SA[1,2], Black RE[1], Checkley W[1]

[1]Department of International Health, Bloomberg School of Public Health, The Johns Hopkins University, Baltimore, MD, USA; [2]Fogarty International Center, National Institutes of Health, Bethesda, MD, USA

Adv Nutr 2012; 3: 250–254

Background: Although progress is being made in decreasing undernutrition in low- and middle-income countries, wasting (weight-for-height z-score <−2) and stunting (height-for-age z-score <−2) during childhood continue to burden the poorest regions in the developing world. Ponderal and linear growth of children has been widely studied. However, epidemiologic evidence of a relationship between the two is inconsistent. Understanding the relationship between weight-for-height and height-for-age will allow organizations to better design and evaluate programs to improve childhood nutrition.

Results: At a cross-sectional level, there appears to be a limited relationship between ponderal and linear growth. Individual level, cross-sectional studies have found little association between weight-for-height and height-for-age. Cross-sectional, population-level studies have demonstrated that height for age decreases throughout the first 2–3 years of life in many developing countries, whereas weight-for-height tends to falter during a more limited age window in the first year of life, after which weight-for-height stabilizes or increases. The precise timing of the weight-for-height faltering varies according to the country-specific age of weaning and other local factors. The geographic differences observed in linear and ponderal growth are most probably due to a combination of factors, including maternal nutritional status, exposure to and treatment of infectious diseases as well as dietary factors. If a child has an acute illness or dietary deficiency that result in weight loss, linear growth may slow down or cease until weight is recovered. Once the child regains weight, linear growth will continue and, given adequate nutritional resources and no further infections, catch-up growth may occur, returning the child to the original growth trajectory. However, children in developing countries often experience multiple insults with limited recovery time, leading to persistent height deficits.

Conclusions: Decreased weight-for-height and height-for-age are both important risk factors for illness and death during childhood, and changes in weight appear to have a lagged effect on height during early childhood. Further research is needed to identify the factors associated with recovery of linear growth after a child experiences an insult with decreased weight-for-height. A better understanding of these relationships will enable program managers to design improved strategies to intervene in order to improve childhood nutrition, growth and health.

Comments   In the present review the authors discuss the interpretation of different variables of the growth charts and the relationships between them. It is an important paper since it highlights the strength and limitations of growth charts and the information that can be derived and used from such data both on different populations and on an individual child. About 200 million children under the age of 5 in the developing world are stunted, most likely due to inadequate nutrition, and suffer from repeated episodes of infectious diseases. The growth chart is a very important tool for the pediatrician when following an individual child and for health authorities when following pediatric populations. Understanding the relationships between height-for-age, weight-for-age and weight-for-height in developing countries and their changes during intervention programs are extremely important and should be studied in prospective studies since better and cheaper tools for assessing nutritional interventions in different parts of the world do not exist.

Linear growth and final height characteristics in adolescent females with anorexia nervosa

Modan-Moses D[1,3], Yaroslavsky A[2], Kochavi B[2], Toledano A[2], Segev S[2], Balawi F[2], Mitrany E[2], Stein D[2,3]

[1]Pediatric Endocrinology and Diabetes Unit, The Edmond and Lily Safra Children's Hospital, The Chaim Sheba Medical Center, Tel-Hashomer, Ramat Gan, Israel; [2]Pediatric Psychosomatic Department, The Edmond and Lily Safra Children's Hospital, The Chaim Sheba Medical Center, Tel-Hashomer, Ramat Gan, Israel; [3]The Sackler School of Medicine, Tel Aviv University, Tel Aviv, Israel

PLoS One 2012; 7: e45504

Objective: Malnutrition often results in growth deceleration, while nutritional rehabilitation results in catch-up growth that is often incomplete, resulting in compromised final adult height. Anorexia nervosa (AN) provides a model for studying the effect of caloric restriction during adolescence on growth and final height. Several studies reported growth failure or short stature in patients with AN. However, data regarding final height of patients with AN is scarce and inconclusive. The aims of the study were to evaluate the prevalence of growth retardation in a cohort of female adolescent patients with AN in order to assess the effect of weight restoration on catch-up growth and final height and to identify factors affecting catch-up growth and final height.

Methods: All female patients with AN (n = 211), hospitalized in an inpatient eating disorders department from January 1, 1987 to December 31, 1999, were included in this study and their medical charts were retrospectively reviewed. After assessment of the nutritional status, a nutritional rehabilitation program geared toward weight gain of 0.5–1.0 kg/week was constructed. Target weight was established according to age and the estimated potential height. Patients were discharged upon reaching their target weight and maintaining it for at least 2 weeks. After discharge, patients were followed until reaching the age of 18. Target weight was readjusted every 3 months during follow-up in patients who had not finished growing, and was increased gradually to allow for the expected height gain, based on the potential height. Height and weight were assessed at admission and thereafter routinely during hospitalization and follow-up. Final height (defined as height at age 18 or older, and at least 3 years after menarche) was measured in 69 patients 2–10 years after discharge.

Results: The mean age of the patients on admission was 16.6 ± 4.2 years; their mean BMI was 15.7 ± 1.02, and their mean age at menarche was 12.7 ± 2.4 years. Patients' height standard deviation scores (SDS) on admission (–0.285 ± 1.02) and discharge (–0.271 ± 1.02) were significantly lower than expected in normal adolescents (p < 0.001). The extent of growth impairment was more severe among patients admitted at the age of ≤13 years on both admission and discharge than patients admitted at an older age (p = 0.03), and patients admitted less than 1 year after menarche had more severe growth impairment on admission than patients admitted more than 1 year after menarche (height SDS –0.38 ± 1.01 vs. –0.19 ± 0.92, p = 0.03). Final height SDS, available for 69 patients, was –0.258 ± 1.04, significantly lower than expected in a normal population (p = 0.04), and was more severely compromised in patients who were admitted less than 1 year from their menarche. Height SDS on admission was a strong predictor of final height SDS (p < 0.001). BMI-SDS upon admission was negatively correlated with the change in height SDS between admission and final height (r = –0.306, p = 0.011). Other factors, including weight gain during hospitalization, duration of hospitalization, number of hospitalizations, and duration of AN prior to hospitalization had no significant effect on final height SDS. Complete growth data (i.e. pre-morbid, admission, discharge, and final height) was available for 29 patients. In these patients the pre-morbid height SDS was not significantly different from the expected (–0.11 ± 1.1), whereas heights at the other time points were significantly lower (–0.56 ± 1.2, –0.52 ± 1.2, and –0.6 ± 1.2, respectively, p = 0.001).

Conclusions: The findings of the study show that whereas the pre-morbid height of female adolescent with AN is normal, linear growth retardation is a prominent feature of the illness. Weight restoration is associated with catch-up growth, but complete catch-up is often not achieved with impaired final height. The findings emphasize the importance of early detection of AN, as growth retardation occurring during a critical growth period during puberty may be irreversible. Weight restoration geared towards restitution of height to the pre-morbid percentile for age should be initiated as early as possible.

Comments This is a relatively large study that assesses the effect of undernutrition during puberty on growth rate and final adult height AN provides an opportunity to study the 'pure' interaction between nutrition and growth in the adolescent age group since AN is not associated with other diseases which might affect growth, such as malnutrition in the developing countries. Adolescent girls with AN do catch-up during nutritional rehabilitation despite the fact that they usually present at a relatively 'old' age (mean age 16.6 ± 4.2 years). It is an important study despite the fact that it is of retrospective nature, thus it is associated with many limitations. It is possible that earlier admission could have a better outcome despite the authors' observation that patients admitted under the age of 13 years or less than 1 year after menarche were more severely affected than patients admitted at an older age. It is possible that patients who were admitted in an earlier age where more severely affected by the disease already at its earlier stages and started their AN at an earlier age than the patients who were admitted at an older age. It is clear that a prospective study is crucial to better understand the interaction between nutrition and growth in the adolescent age group using AN as a model. In such a study, information on the age when first symptoms appear, previous growth data, bone age, parents' height and family history should be collected and analyzed and the 'best' rehabilitation program should be studied. A well-designed study could potentially teach us more about the interaction between nutrition and growth than any large retrospective study.

Catch-up growth after long-term implementation and weaning from ketogenic diet in pediatric epileptic patients

Kim JT[1], Kang H-C[1], Song J-E[1], Lee MJ[1], Lee YJ[2], Lee EJ[3], Lee JS[1], Kim HD[1]

[1]Division of Pediatric Neurology, Department of Pediatrics, Pediatric Epilepsy Clinic, Severance Children's Hospital, Epilepsy Research Institute, Yonsei University College of Medicine, Seoul, Republic of Korea; [2]Department of Pediatrics, Pusan National University Children's Hospital, Pusan National University School of Medicine, Yangsan, Republic of Korea; [3]Division of Dietetics, Severance Hospital, Yonsei University College of Medicine, Seoul, Republic of Korea

Clin Nutr 2013; 32: 98–103

Objective: Ketogenic diet (KD) is a potent, accepted treatment in childhood epilepsy resistant to other medications. Previous studies have reported significant reductions in height and weight gain among children after implementation of KD. However, long-term studies on growth following discontinuation of long-term KD are still lacking. The aim was to analyze the presence of growth delay among children with epilepsy during implementation of long-term KD, and to assess the presence of catch-up growth 1 year after diet discontinuation.

Methods: Data were retrospectively collected from chart review of 40 children (20 males) with intractable epilepsy who began long-term KD, followed by successful weaning after more than 2 years of diet implementation. Inclusion criteria consisted of follow-up at the outpatient clinic with well-documented epidemiologic and clinical data (including height and weight measurements) at the onset of the KD, 2 years with the diet, and 1 year after weaning. Growth retardation was defined as a statistically significant drop in mean z-scores of clinical parameter as compared to baseline. If growth retardation was followed by return to baseline z-scores or was followed by significant increase in z-scores of the clinical parameters after diet discontinuation, it was considered as catch-up growth.

Results: The median age at seizure onset was 0.79 ± 3.31 years (range 0.01–10.67), and the median age at start of KD was 4.58 ± 5.29 years (range 0.58–15.52). Subjects continued the diet for a mean duration of 2.35 ± 0.36 years (range 2.00–3.26). Mean period of follow-up after the diet was 1.70 ± 0.43 years (range 1.00–2.42). A significant reduction was found in both height and weight gain after prolonged KD. After a year of diet discontinuation, significant catch-up growth was evident in both height and weight. When comparing the growth patterns among subsets of the study patients, ambulation had favorable influence on growth during KD and after diet discontinuation. Uncontrolled epilepsy and younger age at the start of KD contributed a negative impact on growth pattern.

Conclusions: KD is an effective treatment modality in intractable epileptic patients, and decreased growth velocity is a risk that most patients and guardians are willing to take. This preliminary study of long-term growth pattern among children treated with KD will aid in planning for long-term care extending beyond the duration of dietary treatment.

Comments   In recent years, the use of KD to treat patients with retractable epilepsy regained popularity among physicians since its effectiveness was shown to exceed in some cases even to most modern medications. The effect of KD on weight and height was described in the literature before but the present study allows us to get information of children's growth with the use of currently used KD protocols. The authors confirmed that indeed the use of KD for 2 years interferes with weight and height gain of children in different age groups. There was a significant reduction in height and weight z score after 2 years on DK with a statistical improvement in these parameters after a year of regular diet.

It is an important study even though the number of patients studied was small and the follow-up period was limited (only 1 year on 'regular diet') since it confirms previous observations of attenuated growth during KD and suggests catch-up growth thereafter. However, it does not shed light on the mechanism by which KD influences growth and therefore does not contribute to our understanding of the mechanism of that phenomenon. It also does not teach us which diet was used during the year of catch-up. It seems like 2 years of KD is safe in most age groups since catch-up does occur during the year following the intervention period (except for the young age group) but what is the longest 'safe' period of KD in the different pediatric age groups? In addition, only 1 year of follow-up after KD was documented. The present study confirms the need for a prospective study with more patients and for a longer period of time in order to better understand the long-term effect of KD in the pediatric age group.

Catch-up growth in children born growth-restricted to mothers with hypertensive disorders of pregnancy

Beukers F[1], Cranendonk A[2], de Vries JIP[3], Wolf H[4], Lafeber HN[2], Vriesendorp HC[1], Ganzevoort W[4], van Wassenaer-Leemhuis AG[1]

[1]Department of Neonatology, Academic Medical Center, Amsterdam, The Netherlands;
[2]Department of Neonatology, VU University Medical Center, Amsterdam, The Netherlands;
[3]Department of Obstetrics and Gynaecology, VU University Medical Center, Amsterdam, The Netherlands; [4]Department of Obstetrics and Gynaecology, Academic Medical Center, Amsterdam, The Netherlands

Arch Dis Child 2013; 98: 30–35

Background: Fetal growth restriction (FGR) occurs frequently in preterm hypertensive disorders of pregnancy. This may vary in different regions and have long-term implications. The authors examined growth prospectively in a cohort of 135 children born to mothers who were admitted before 34 weeks' gestational age with a severe hypertensive disorder of pregnancy and evaluated height, weight, body mass index (BMI), head circumference (HC), SD scores (SDS) at 3 months and 1 and 4.5 years of age, and complete catch-up growth (height SDS-target height SDS >−1.6).

Results: The investigators found that on average growth scores were lower compared to Dutch growth curves, except for BMI at 3 months and girls' HC at all ages. Mean height SDS increased over time from −1.4 to −0.5 at 4.5 years, with 94% having complete catch-up growth. Mean BMI SDS also decreased from −0.2 at 3 months to −1.0 at 1 year, and was −0.8 at age 4.5. Mean HC SDS did not change over time and −0.3 at 4.5 years.

Conclusion: The authors concluded that although the majority of children born growth-restricted had catch-up growth of height within the normal range at 4.5 years of age, they remained smaller and lighter compared to Dutch growth charts. The customized birth weight ratio, as a measure of the degree of FGR, was related to all growth SDS at 4.5 years, while no association was seen with prematurity expressed by gestational age at birth.

Comments The finding that fetal growth restriction or intrauterine growth retardation was associated with long-term effects on linear growth and body size is well recognized and reported across various countries and contexts. In a recent analysis of factors affecting growth across the world [4], close to 20% of all stunting at 24 months of age was attributed to being born small for gestational age (SGA). The fact that the degree of FGR was associated with all growth outcomes among the Dutch growth cohort is consistent with these observations and confirms the association. Recent data [5] also confirm the association of prematurity and fetal growth retardation in a subset of newborn infants in various geographies. The authors did not study this prematurity-SGA interaction which might have been of interest. There is also no information provided on metabolic factors or body composition at any of the time points and hence it is difficult to comment on associations with body fat distribution with status at birth or varying patterns of linear growth and catch-up in infancy and early childhood. The association of long-term outcomes with patterns of linear growth in early childhood is well recognized [6] and one hopes that this particular cohort would also be tracked to adult life.

Health profile of young adults born preterm: negative effects of rapid weight gain in early life

Kerkhof GF, Willemsen RH, Leunissen RW, Breukhoven PE, Hokken-Koelega AC

Department of Pediatrics, Subdivision of Endocrinology, Erasmus Medical Center/Sophia Children's Hospital, GJ Rotterdam, The Netherlands

J Clin Endocrinol Metab 2012; 97: 4498–4506

Background: The association of early postnatal weight gain with risks of developing cardiovascular disease (CVD) and type 2 diabetes mellitus (DM2) in adults born at term is well recognized. However, relatively little is known of such risks in infants born preterm. The authors investigated the association of weight gain and weight trajectories during early childhood among infants born prematurely with determinants of CVD and DM2 in early adulthood; specifically they assessed growth in infancy and determinants of CVD and DM2 among 162 young adults (18–24 years) born preterm (gestational age <36 weeks) in comparison with data of 217 young adults born at term.

Results: The authors demonstrated that early gain in weight for length in the period from preterm birth up to term and the 3 months thereafter was positively correlated with % body fat, waist circumference, total cholesterol and low-density lipoprotein cholesterol levels at 21 years of age. These effects were more marked in subjects with the highest weight gain in weight from birth to term age and rapid catch-up in weight thereafter in the first 3 months had significantly higher body fat percentage, waist circumference, acute insulin response and disposition index in early adulthood than subgroups with moderate and slower catch-up in weight.

Conclusions: The authors concluded that accelerated neonatal gain in weight relative to length after preterm birth (immediately after birth and during the first 3 months after term age) may be associated with metabolic changes suggestive of excessive risk CVD in early adulthood.

Comments These findings present associations of early weight gain in the first few months of life with biomarkers of potential CVD (body fat, waist circumference and lipid levels). Given that linear growth data were not a focus of attention and that 'rapid growth' was largely defined as gains in weight and weight for length, it is difficult to ascertain the subset who gained in both length and weight ('optimal growth'). Early weight gain in the first 2 years of life has been shown to be appropriate and safe in evaluation of long-term outcomes in multi-country cohorts [7] and linear growth has been shown to be of benefit in recent evaluations based on pooled analysis of the same populations [6]. These findings must therefore be taken in the context of existing data and further information sought on linear growth as well as growth patterns in the 0- to 24-month window to assess the validity of this association. The issues in relation to the lack of information on patterns of intrauterine growth and standards are valid and could well be resolved by availability of intrauterine growth standards from the Intergrowth 21st study later this year.

Associated factors for accelerated growth in childhood: a systematic review

Chrestani MA[1], Santos IS[1], Horta BL[1], Dumith SC[2], de Oliveira Dode MA[1]

[1]Federal University of Pelotas, Pelotas, Brazil; [2]Federal University of Rio Grande (FURG), Rio Grande, RS, Brazil

Matern Child Health J 2013; 17: 512–519

Background: The authors conducted a systematic review of factors associated with accelerated growth, or catch-up growth based on studies (English, Spanish or Portuguese) in the Medline/PubMed database. The term 'catch-up' has been used for the accelerated growth of children who have suffered from restricted intrauterine growth based on either maternal nutritional factors or morbidity such as hypertensive disease. The authors focused on studies of outcomes in children 0–12 years of age who had either accelerated growth or catch-up growth studied after birth.
Results: There was a remarkable paucity of literature and out of the 2,155 articles highlighted, only 9 were considered suitable for further study. The authors found no uniformity in the operational definition of accelerated growth, or in the concept of catch-up. Factors associated with accelerated growth included primiparity, maternal smoking during pregnancy, lower birth weight, and early weaning.
Conclusions: The authors identified major limitations in the studies as lack of adequate controls and high rates of loss to follow-up. They called for further studies as they were unable to find convincing risk factors associated with accelerated growth in the available literature.

Comments This review is illustrative of the state of the current evidence around early child growth and development with relatively few prospective observational studies and trials. As evidenced by data from the COHORTS studies, there is paucity of information on intrauterine and postnatal growth patterns, especially in relation to gestational age. The latter has been difficult to standardize in studies based on recall of maternal menstrual dates and expected date of delivery. Improvements in technology, notably ultrasound assessment of gestational age, have made it possible to assess fetal maturity with confidence and also assess phenotypes with a greater degree of confidence [8, 9]. Future studies also need to include biomarkers [10] in addition to growth and development parameters.

J.H. and J.B. statement: Acknowledgement: This work was supported in part by the Intramural Research Program of the Eunice Kennedy Shriver National Institute of Child Health and Human Development (NICHD).

References

1 Emma F, Sesto A, Rizzoni G: Long-term linear growth of children with severe steroid-responsive nephrotic syndrome. Pediatr Nephrol 2003;18:783–788.

2 Chevalley T, Bonjour JP, Ferrari S, Rizzoli R: The influence of pubertal timing on bone mass acquisition: a predetermined trajectory detectable five years before menarche. J Clin Endocrinol Metab 2009;94:3424–3431.

3 Teilmann G, Petersen JH, Gormsen M, Damgaard K, Skakkebaek NE, Jensen TK: Early puberty in internationally adopted girls: hormonal and clinical markers of puberty in 276 girls examined biannually over two years. Horm Res 2009;72:236–246.

4 Black RE, Victora CG, Walker SP, Bhutta ZA, Christian P, de Onis M, Ezzati M, Grantham-McGregor S, Katz J, Martorell R, Uauy R, Maternal and Child Nutrition Study Group: Maternal and child undernutrition and overweight in low-income and middle-income countries. Lancet 2013;382:427–451.

5 Katz J, Lee AC, Kozuki N, Lawn JE, Cousens S, Blencowe H, Ezzati M, Bhutta ZA, Marchant T, Willey BA, Adair L, Barros F, Baqui AH, Christian P, Fawzi W, Gonzalez R, Humphrey J, Huybregts L, Kolsteren P, Mongkolchati A, Mullany LC, Ndyomugyenyi R, Nien JK, Osrin D, Roberfroid D, Sania A, Schmiegelow C, Silveira MF, Tielsch J, Vaidya A, Velaphi SC, Victora CG, Watson-Jones D, Black RE, CHERG Small-for-Gestational-Age-Preterm Birth Working Group: Mortality risk in preterm and small-for-gestational-age infants in low-income and middle-income countries: a pooled country analysis. Lancet 2013;382:417–425.

6 Adair LS, Fall CH, Osmond C, Stein AD, Martorell R, Ramirez-Zea M, Sachdev HS, Dahly DL, Bas I, Norris SA, Micklesfield L, Hallal P, Victora CG, COHORTS group: Associations of linear growth and relative weight gain during early life with adult health and human capital in countries of low and middle income: findings from five birth cohort studies. Lancet 2013;382:525–534.

7 Victora CG, Adair L, Fall C, Hallal PC, Martorell R, Richter L, Sachdev HS, Maternal and Child Undernutrition Study Group: Maternal and child undernutrition: consequences for adult health and human capital. Lancet 2008;371:340–357.

8 Villar J, Papageorghiou AT, Knight HE, Gravett MG, Iams J, Waller SA, Kramer M, Culhane JF, Barros FC, Conde-Agudelo A, Bhutta ZA, Goldenberg RL: The preterm birth syndrome: a prototype phenotypic classification. Am J Obstet Gynecol 2012;206:119–123.

9 Goldenberg RL, Gravett MG, Iams J, Papageorghiou AT, Waller SA, Kramer M, Culhane J, Barros F, Conde-Agudelo A, Bhutta ZA, Knight HE, Villar J: The preterm birth syndrome: issues to consider in creating a classification system. Am J Obstet Gynecol 2012;206:113–118.

10 Conde-Agudelo A, Papageorghiou AT, Kennedy SH, Villar J: Novel biomarkers for the prediction of the spontaneous preterm birth phenotype: a systematic review and meta-analysis. BJOG 2011;118:1042–1054.

Koletzko B, Shamir R, Turck D, Phillip M (eds): Nutrition and Growth: Yearbook 2014.
World Rev Nutr Diet. Basel, Karger, 2014, vol 109, pp 101–108 (DOI: 10.1159/000356110)

Pregnancy: Impact of Maternal Nutrition on Intrauterine Fetal Growth

Yariv Yogev[1,2] and Liran Hiersch[1,2]

[1] Helen Schneider Hospital for Women, Rabin Medical Center, Petach-Tikva, Israel
[2] The Sackler Faculty of Medicine, Tel Aviv University, Tel Aviv, Israel

This chapter of the *Yearbook on Nutrition and Growth* reviews important articles published between July 2012 and July 2013 concerning the impact of maternal nutrition during pregnancy on intrauterine fetal growth. Along with human studies, several animal studies dealing with the effect of nutrition on the placenta are also included since this field is not sufficiently studied in humans. Finally, we included future studies that hopefully will help in understanding the goals and interventional options for healthier offspring.

Human Studies

Low glycaemic index diet in pregnancy to prevent macrosomia (ROLO study): randomised control trial

Walsh JM, McGowan CA, Mahony R, Foley ME, McAuliffe FM

UCD Obstetrics and Gynaecology, School of Medicine and Medical Science, University College Dublin, National Maternity Hospital, Dublin, Ireland
BMJ 2012; 345: e5605

Background: Pregnancies associated with large for gestational age and macrosomia fetuses are at increased risk for adverse maternal and neonatal outcome such as birth complications and obesity later in the offspring's life compared to those with appropriate for gestational age fetuses. The objective of the current study was to determine whether a low glycaemic index diet in pregnancy could reduce the incidence of macrosomia in an at-risk group.
Methods: Between January 2007 and January 2011, 800 non-diabetic pregnant women in their second pregnancy prior to 18 weeks of gestation with previous newborns weighing >4 kg were randomized to either no dietary intervention or low glycaemic index diet. The primary outcome measure was difference in birth weight. The secondary outcome measure was difference in maternal gestational weight gain.

Results: Regarding the primary outcome, no significant difference was seen between the two groups in absolute birth weight, birth weight centile, or ponderal index. However, regarding the secondary outcome, significantly less gestational weight gain occurred in women in the intervention arm. The rate of glucose intolerance was also lower in the intervention arm: 21% compared with 28% of controls had a fasting glucose ≥5.1 mmol/l or a 1-hour glucose challenge test result ≥7.8 mmol/l.

Conclusion: In a risk group for macrosomia, a low glycaemic index diet in pregnancy did not reduce the incidence of large for gestational age infants. It did, however, have a significant positive effect on gestational weight gain and maternal glucose intolerance.

Comments According to the World Health Organization (WHO), over 600 million adults worldwide are clinically obese. With the growing knowledge of the association between large for gestational age and obesity later in life, effective strategies in order to halt this problem are needed. The current study is a sufficiently powered randomized control trial. Several interventional studies in the past reported that a low glycemic index diet is useful in reducing birth weight and the prevalence of large for gestational age infants. Those studies, however, had a small sample size compared to the current study. Moreover, in previous studies a much more intense regimen of intervention was used, whereas in the current study there were only a few reinforcing meetings throughout pregnancy. Women in the intervention group had gained in average 1.5 kg less than those in the control group. This relatively minor reduction of weight gain was successful in reducing the rate of glucose intolerance. Perhaps a diet that could accomplish even less weight gain during pregnancy would help in reducing birth weight infants as well.

The Mediterranean diet and fetal size parameters: the Generation R Study

Timmermans S[1,2], Steegers-Theunissen RP[2-5], Vujkovic M[2], den Breeijen H[3], Russcher H[6], Lindemans J[6], Mackenbach J[7], Hofman A[3], Lesaffre EE[8,9], Jaddoe VV[1,3,4], Steegers EA[2]

[1]Generation R Study Group, Erasmus Medical Center, Rotterdam, The Netherlands; [2]Department of Obstetrics and Gynecology, Erasmus Medical Center, Rotterdam, The Netherlands; [3]Department of Epidemiology, Erasmus Medical Center, Rotterdam, The Netherlands; [4]Department of Pediatrics, Erasmus Medical Center, Rotterdam, The Netherlands; [5]Department of Clinical Genetics, Erasmus Medical Center, Rotterdam, The Netherlands; [6]Department of Clinical Chemistry, Erasmus Medical Center, Rotterdam, The Netherlands; [7]Department of Public Health, Erasmus Medical Center, Rotterdam, The Netherlands; [8]Department of Biostatistics, Erasmus Medical Center, Rotterdam, The Netherlands, and [9]Biostatistical Centre, Catholic University Leuven, Leuven, Belgium

Br J Nutr 2012; 108: 1399–1409

Background: Developmental adaptations due to early nutritional exposures may have permanent health consequences. Up to date, most studies exploring the association between maternal nutrition and fetal size have mainly focused on individual nutrients. The current study focused on the pattern of food consumption and its significance.

Methods: A prospective observational study was conducted between 2001 and 2006. The present analysis was restricted to 3,207 prenatally enrolled Dutch women with a spontaneously conceived, live-born singleton pregnancy. Participants completed a semiquantitative questionnaire during early (gestational age <18 weeks) pregnancy evaluating their diet habits. Logistic regression analysis was used to predict the occurrence of intrauterine growth retardation at birth as a function of food intake. The derived solution was considered as the dietary pattern. A combination of higher intakes of fruit, vegetables, vegetable oil, fish, pasta and rice, and lower intakes of meat, potatoes and fatty sauces was labeled the 'Mediterranean' diet. The study evaluated the association of dietary habits with fetal size, uteroplacental vascular resistance, placental weight and birth weight.

Results: Fetal size and placental parameters were associated with the degree of adherence to Mediterranean diet. Women with low adherence to the diet had a 72 g lower birth weight and a 15 g lower placental weight compared to women with high adherence to the diet. No difference regarding uteroplacental vascular resistance was observed between the studied groups.

Conclusion: Low adherence to a Mediterranean diet in early pregnancy seems to be associated with a lower placental mass and a lower birth weight.

Comments Over the past years, the Mediterranean diet has gained popularity for its positive health effects. While no single Mediterranean diet exists, dietary patterns that prevail in the Mediterranean region share common characteristics including high intakes of vegetables and vegetables oil, moderate amounts of fish and a relatively low consumption of meat. Although showing only a modest effect on infant and placental weight, the current study is important as being one of the first studies to examine the relationship between dietary habits in early pregnancy (as opposed to a specific micronutrient) and fetal and placental growth during intrauterine life. The result of the current study supports previous reports of a reduced rate of intrauterine growth restriction fetuses associated with a dietary pattern rich in fruits and vegetables compared with one rich in meat, snacks and potatoes.

Dietary balance during pregnancy is associated with fetal adiposity and fat distribution

Blumfield ML[1,3], Hure AJ[2,3], MacDonald-Wicks LK[1], Smith R[2,3], Simpson SJ[4], Giles WB[5], Raubenheime D[6], Collins CE[1,3]

[1]The School of Health Sciences, Faculty of Health, University of Newcastle, Callaghan, NSW, Australia; [2]The School of Medicine and Public Health, Faculty of Health, University of Newcastle, Callaghan, NSW, Australia; [3]The Mothers and Babies Research Centre, Hunter Medical Research Institute, John Hunter Hospital, NSW, Australia; [4]The School of Biological Sciences, Northern Clinical School, [5]Obstetrics, Gynaecology and Neonatology, Northern Clinical School, [6]University of Sydney, Sydney, NSW, Australia, and The Institute of Natural Sciences, Massey University, Albany, New Zealand

Am J Clin Nutr 2012; 96: 1032–1041

Background: The in utero environment could affect the offspring phenotype. Lean body composition at birth is associated with an increased risk for subsequent cardiac and metabolic illness in adulthood.

Methods: The study prospectively assessed 179 Australian women with singleton pregnancies from the Women and Their Children's Health (WATCH) Study. Maternal diet was quantified by a validated food-frequency questionnaire at 18–24 and 36–40 weeks of gestation. Fetal body composition measurements were ascertained from abdominal and midthigh sites by ultrasound performed at 19, 25, 30, and 36 weeks.

Results: Maternal intakes of protein and starch and the protein:carbohydrate ratio was associated with the percentage of abdominal fat, whereas saturated fatty acids (SFA) and polyunsaturated fatty acid (PUFA) were associated with the percentage of midthigh fat. Fetal adiposity was maximized at different macronutrient intakes. Abdominal fat was highest with low protein intakes and midthigh fat was highest at intermediate protein, high fat (>40% of energy) and low carbohydrate (<40% of energy) intakes.

Conclusion: Fetal body fat composition may be modifiable via nutritional intervention in the mother.

Comments   In contrast to the previous studies presented above addressing infant weight, the current study deals with the association between maternal nutrition during pregnancy and fetal body composition. It was suggested in the past that fetal small abdominal viscera and low muscle mass but a preserved proportion of body fat is associated with insulin resistance later in life. However, the ideal neonatal body composition, which would be associated with optimal short- and long-term outcome, is yet to be determined, and also whether this 'idealism' is related to the infant total weight. It is interesting that the effect of maternal macronutrient profile was different between fetal abdominal and midthigh sites. Unfortunately, direct measurement of neonatal adiposity at birth was not performed; thus, a correlation between the sonographic and the actual measurement could not be established.

Plasma lipids and lipoproteins during pregnancy and related pregnancy outcomes

Emet T, Ustüner I, Güven SG, Balık G, Ural UM, Tekin YB, Sentürk S, Sahin FK, Avşar AF

Department of Obstetrics and Gynecology, Recep Tayyip Erdoğan University School of Medicine, Rize, Turkey

Arch Gynecol Obstet 2013 (E-pub ahead of print)

Background: During pregnancy, complex changes occur in lipid metabolism. Increased lipid synthesis and maternal hyperphagia lead to fat accumulation especially in the first and second trimesters. This process is reversed during the third trimester due to increased lipolytic activity in the adipose tissue. The aim of the current study was to explore the association between maternal changes in lipid profile with pregnancy outcome.

Methods: In a prospective study, 1,000 pregnant women were recruited in the years 2010–2011. Lipid profile tests including triglyceride (TG), total cholesterol, high-density lipoprotein (HDL) and low-density lipoprotein (LDL) were established in the first antenatal visit (<14 weeks) and repeated in the third trimester (>28 weeks). The maternal nutritional as well as medical and social-demographic status was recorded. Primary outcome measures were defined as the association of the pregnancy-related lipid profile change to neonatal weight, the weight of the infant in the third month and pregnancy complications.

Results: The levels of TG, total cholesterol, HDL and LDL increased significantly as pregnancy progressed. Patients with good nutritional parameters had the higher percentage of change in the TG levels. An increased percentage of change in the TG levels had a positive effect on neonatal weight, but not on the placental weight and the third month weight of the infant. An inverse relation was observed between the percent change in TG levels and the risk of the preterm birth.

Conclusion: In pregnancy, complex alterations occur in lipid metabolism. Percent change in TG levels is positively affected by the maternal nutrition level. The neonatal weight and the risk of preterm birth are affected by the percent change in TG levels.

Comments   The purpose of the current study was to explore the effect of maternal lipid profile changes in pregnancy in relation to fetal growth and development, prognosis, and complications of pregnancy. The current study result joins previous reports regarding the increase in lipid levels during pregnancy. The main difference of this work in comparison to previous studies was the assessment of the percentile change in lipid profile between early and late gestation and its effect on pregnancy outcome. Therefore, lipid profile should be assessed several times during pregnancy as a single measurement could be misleading. Maternal nutritional status showed an association only to the change in TG levels and not to other parameters of the lipid profile. A possible future implication for this finding is that the change in TG levels during pregnancy may assist in evaluating maternal nutritional status. Moreover, this parameter was associated to both neonatal weight and the risk of preterm birth.

Maternal nutrition and birth outcomes: effect of balanced protein-energy supplementation

Imdad A, Bhutta ZA

Division of Women and Child Health, Aga Khan University, Karachi, Pakistan
Paediatr Perinat Epidemiol 2012; 26: 178–190

Summary: This paper reviews the evidence on the association of maternal nutrition with birth outcome and the effect of balanced protein-energy supplementation (protein provides <25% of total energy content) in particular. Sixteen intervention studies were included in the review. Only randomized, quasi-randomized trials and before-after designs were included. Pooled analysis showed a positive impact of balanced protein-energy supplementation on birth weight compared with control. Protein-energy supplementation was associated with a reduced rate of low birth weight infants and a reduced risk for intrauterine growth restriction. The effect was more pronounced in undernourished women compared with adequately nourished women.

Comments   This is a meta-analysis regarding the association of balanced protein-energy supplementation and fetal weight. The strength of this study is the inclusion of interventional studies only. In any case, subgroup analyses based on the nutritional status of the mothers showed that balanced protein-energy supplementation was more effective in malnourished women than adequately nourished ones. However, there were no standardized criteria to define undernourished women. Moreover, none of the studies used body mass index (BMI) as the recruitment criteria. A similar evaluation was conducted by the Cochrane review. However, while the Cochrane review results were in accordance with the current study results, the results of the current analysis reached statistical significance (as opposed to the Cochrane review) mainly due to the inclusion of 5 more studies in the current analysis which provided its statistical magnitude.

Animal Studies

Effect of maternal dietary energy types on placenta nutrient transporter gene expressions and intrauterine fetal growth in rats

Lin Y, Zhuo Y, Fang ZF, Che LQ, Wu D

Key Laboratory for Animal Disease Resistance Nutrition, Ministry of Education, and Animal Nutrition Institute, Sichuan Agricultural University, Ya'an, PR China
Nutrition 2012; 28: 1037–1043

Background: The mechanism mediating the maternal nutritional effects on fetal growth is unclear. Intrauterine growth is largely determined by the capacity of the placenta to supply nutrients from the mother to the fetus which depends primarily on the function of the placental nutrient transporter. The investigators wished to explore the effect of different maternal energy-intake types on placental nutrient transporters and whether fetal growth could be associated with different gene expressions relating to fetal DNA methylation and energy metabolism.

Methods: Three-month-old rats (n = 72) were allocated to one of four groups: low fat/low fiber (L-L), low fat/high fiber (L-H), high fat/low fiber (H-L), or high fat/high fiber (H-H). Rats were fed the treatment diets 4 weeks before mating and continued in pregnancy until sample collections were obtained on days 13.5 and 17.5 of pregnancy.

Results: The fetal weight in the L-L group was significantly lower than that in the H-L group. The placental nutrient transporter mRNA expressions of glucose transporter-3 (Slc2a3) and cationic amino acid transporter-1 (Slc7a1) in the L-L group with a decreased fetal weight were downregulated compared with that in the H-L group with an increased fetal weight. For the placental imprinted gene Igf-2 and H19 expressions, lower Igf-2 and higher H19 expressions were associated with the decreased fetal growth in the L-L group compared with the H-L group with an increased fetal weight. A different fetal growth was associated with different DNA methyltransferase-1 and methyltransferase-3a expressions and energy metabolism-related genes.

Conclusion: Different energy-intake types could affect intrauterine fetal growth and it is regulated through placental nutrient transporter gene expressions.

Comments   The placenta plays a crucial role in the growth and the survival of the fetus in utero. This study not only explored the association between different energy-intake types on the fetal growth, but also reported on the placental role in this process. Moreover, they showed that there is alternation in gene expression in both the placenta and the fetus in response to maternal diet. However, while those genomic adaptations could be important for fetal survival in utero, it is possible that this mal-programing in genes associated with fetal metabolism could be responsible for an adverse metabolic outcome later in the offspring life.

Maternal calorie restriction modulates placental mitochondrial biogenesis and bioenergetic efficiency: putative involvement in fetoplacental growth defects in rats

Mayeur S, Lancel S, Theys N, Lukaszewski MA, Duban-Deweer S, Bastide B, Hachani J, Cecchelli R, Breton C, Gabory A, Storme L, Reusens B, Junien C, Vieau D, Lesage J

Université Lille Nord de France, Lille, France

Am J Physiol Endocrinol Metab 2013; 304: E14–E22

Background: Maternal undernutrition is known to be associated with decreased fetal growth. This is mainly due to placental inability to supply adequate oxygen and nutrients to the fetus. However, the mechanism by which maternal nutritional status affects the placenta is still unclear.

Methods: Rat term placentas from 70% food-restricted (FR30) mothers were used for a proteomic screen. Placental mitochondrial functions were evaluated using molecular and functional approaches, and ATP production was measured.

Results: FR30 was associated with reduced fetal and placental weight compared with controls. FR30 placentas displayed 14 proteins that were differentially expressed, including several mitochondrial proteins. FR30 induced a marked increase in placental mtDNA content and changes in mitochondrial functions, including modulation of the expression of genes implicated in biogenesis and bioenergetic pathways.

Conclusion: Maternal undernutrition is associated in reduced fetal and placental weight. Fetoplacental pathologies could be explained by placental mitochondrial defects involving biogenesis and bioenergetic pathways.

Comments   The current study explored placental adaptive proteomic processes implicated in response to maternal undernutrition. The main focus of the study was the mitochondrial physiology in the placenta since these organelles play a crucial role in maternofetal exchanges. This is one of the first studies demonstrating the plasticity of the mitochondria in the placenta in response to maternal nutrition. This finding suggests that placental mitochondrial defects could be related to the etiology of intrauterine growth restriction as well.

Future Studies

The objectives, design and implementation of the INTERGROWTH-21st Project

Villar J[1], Altman D[2], Purwar M[3], Noble J[4], Knight H[1], Ruyan P[5], Cheikh Ismail L[1], Barros F[6,7], Lambert A[1], Papageorghiou A[1], Carvalho M[8], Jaffer Y[9], Bertino E[10], Gravett M[11], Bhutta ZA[12], Kennedy S[1], for the International Fetal and Newborn Growth Consortium for the 21st Century (INTERGROWTH-21st)

[1]Nuffield Department of Obstetrics & Gynaecology, and Oxford Maternal & Perinatal Health Institute, Green Templeton College, University of Oxford, Oxford, UK; [2]Centre for Statistics in Medicine, University of Oxford, Oxford, UK; [3]Ketkar Nursing Home, Nagpur, India; [4]Department of Engineering Science, University of Oxford, Oxford, UK; [5]School of Public Health, Peking University, Beijing, China; [6]Programa de Pós-Graduação em Saúde e Comportamento, Universidade Católica de Pelotas, Pelotas, RS, Brazil; [7]Programa de Pós-Graduação em Epidemiologia, Universidade Federal de Pelotas, Pelotas, RS, Brazil; [8]Faculty of Health Sciences, Aga Khan University, Nairobi, Kenya; [9]Department of Family & Community Health, Ministry of Health, Muscat, Sultanate of Oman; [10]Dipartimento di Scienze Pediatriche e dell'Adolescenza, Cattedra di Neonatologia, Università degli Studi di Torino, Torino, Italy; [11]University of Washington School of Medicine, Seattle, WA, USA, and [12]Division of Women & Child Health, The Aga Khan University, Karachi, Pakistan

BJOG 2013 (E-pub ahead of print)

Comments   This is a multicenter, multiethnic, population-based project, being conducted in eight geographical areas. There are 5 objectives to this project. Three sets of international growth standards for (1) fetal growth from early pregnancy, (2) postnatal growth of preterm infants and (3) birth weight, length and head circumference for gestational age. The remaining two objectives are to investigate the determinant of preterm delivery and impaired fetal growth and to develop a prediction model for the estimation of gestational age during mid-trimester based on sonographic measurements. As the project has selected healthy cohorts with no obvious risk factors for intrauterine growth restriction, these standards will describe how all fetuses and newborns should grow, as opposed to traditional charts that describe how some have grown at a given place and time and will allow the identification of at risk population needed for carful surveillance.

The Maternal Obesity Management (MOM) Trial Protocol: a lifestyle intervention during pregnancy to minimize downstream obesity

Adamo KB[1,3,6], Ferraro ZM[1], Goldfield G[1,3,6], Keely E[5,8], Stacey D[4,9], Hadjiyannakis S[1,6,7], Jean-Philippe S[1], Walker M[5,9], Barrowman NJ[2]

[1]Healthy Active Living and Obesity Research Group, Children's Hospital of Eastern Ontario Research Institute, Ottawa, ON, Canada; [2]Children's Hospital of Eastern Ontario Research Institute, Clinical Research Unit Ottawa, ON, Canada; [3]University of Ottawa, Faculty of Health Sciences, School of Human Kinetics, Ottawa, ON, Canada; [4]University of Ottawa, Faculty of Health Sciences, School of Nursing Ottawa, ON, Canada; [5]University of Ottawa, Faculty of Medicine, Obstetrics/Gynecology, Ottawa, ON, Canada; [6]University of Ottawa, Faculty of Medicine, Pediatrics, Ottawa, ON, Canada; [7]Children's Hospital of Eastern Ontario, Centre for Healthy Active Living, Ottawa, ON, Canada; [8]The Ottawa Hospital, Division of Endocrinology and Metabolism, Riverside Campus; Ottawa, ON, Canada; [9]The Ottawa Hospital Research Institute, Centre for Practice Changing Research (CPCR), Ottawa, ON, Canada

Contemp Clin Trials 2013; 35: 87–96

Comments   Pregnancy represents a crucial period both for its effect on the offspring downstream obesity potential and the comorbidity associated with it and as an opportunity in changing maternal behavior since women are highly motivated during that period. This randomized controlled trial objective is to examine whether keeping maternal weight gain during pregnancy within the limits could affect the offspring weight even in long-term follow-up. The MOM trial begins as a pilot study randomizing a total of 60 women in order to examine feasibility and acceptability of the intervention and to provide evidence for future power calculation. Maternal nutrition affects fetal growth in several mechanisms. However, nutrition like any other medical intervention should be personalized taking into consideration the genetic, demographic, behavioral and other factors influencing the potential for fetal growth. In order to achieve that goal, more randomized, well-controlled and adequately powered trials are needed.

Author Index

Schneede, J. 47
Schoendorfer, N.C. 77
Schroder, R. 67
Schuermans, A. 25
Schwab, U. 10
Schwartz, C. 33
Segev, S. 86, 94
Seidel, V. 2
Seidell, J.C. 4
Sentürk, S. 104
Sevilla, A. 37
Shaddy, D.J. 41
Shah, N. 61
Shalitin, S. 1
Shamir, R. IX, 54, 60
Sharma, R. 78
Sharp, N. 77
Sian, L. 30
Sigurdardottir, S. 79
Simmer, K. 43
Simpson, S.J. 103
Slater, A. 39
Smith, R. 103
Smyth, R.L. 69
Soden, S.E. 82
Sommerfelt, H. 47
Song, J.-E. 95
Srinivasan, S. 15
Stacey, D. 108
Standing, J.F. 57
Stanojevic, S. 66
Steegers, E.A. 102
Steegers-Theunissen, R.P. 102
Steer, C.D. 51
Stein, D. 86, 94
Steinbeck, K. 15
Steiner, S.J. 56
Steinman, J. 59
Stephenson, A.L. 66
Stevenson, R.D. 76
Stewart, P.A. 83, 84
Stoltenberg, C. 81
Storme, L. 106
Strain, J.J. 40
Strand, T.A. 47
Sullivan, S. 24
Surén, P. 81
Surveillance of Cerebral Palsy in Europe
    Network 79
Susser, E. 81
Szajewska, H. 26

Taittonen, L. 17
Taneja, S. 47
Taylor, M.A. 27
Tekin, Y.B. 104
Telama, R. 17
Termini, L. 67
Thaker, V. 71
Theys, N. 106
Thodosoff, J.M. 41
Thomas, A. 61
Thorsdottir, I. 32
Tilling, K. 13
Timmermans, S. 102
Toledano, A. 86, 94
Tosh, A.K. 18
Trapnell, B.C. 55
Trauernicht, A. 55
Trauernicht, A.K. 56
Traverso, G. 67
Trawöger, R. 24
Triglia, M.R. 67
Trimarchi, G. 67
Turck, D. IX, 23

Uddenfeldt Wort, U. 78
Ueland, P.M. 47
Uldall, P. 79
Ural, U.M. 104
Ustüner, I. 104

Valéro, R. 85
Van der Hoorn, K. 67
Van der Merwe, L.F. 43
van Goudoever, J.B. 23
Van Rossem, L. 29
van Wassenaer-Leemhuis, A.G. 97
Vanhole, C. 25
Vialettes, B. 85
Vieau, D. 106
Vieni, G. 67
Viikari, J.S.A. 17
Vik, T. 79
Villamor, E. 45, 48
Villar, J. 107
Vitetta, L. 77
Vriesendorp, H.C. 97
Vujkovic, M. 102
Vyncke, K.E. 3

Wagner, P. 78
Walker, J.L. 74, 75, 76

Subject Index

Fetal growth restriction (FGR), catch-up
  growth following hypertensive disorders
  of pregnancy 97
Fish oil, *see* Fatty acids
Folic acid, cognition studies in children
    deficiency effects 47, 48
    maternal status and outcomes 48, 49
    serum concentration correlations 47
Fracture, risk in cerebral palsy 78
FTO, variants and body mass index 10, 11

Gastrostomy
    cerebral palsy management variation across
      Europe 79–81
    cystic fibrosis and nutritional outcomes 70,
      71
    timing in neurodisability 78, 79
Growth hormone (GH)
    resistance in Crohn's disease 55, 56
    therapy for cystic fibrosis 71–74

Hypertension, fetal growth restriction and
  catch-up growth following hypertensive
  disorders of pregnancy 97

Inflammatory bowel disease, *see* Crohn's disease
Insulin-like growth factor-1 (IGF-1), therapy
  for Crohn's disease 57, 58
Iodine, insufficiency in pregnancy and
  cognition 51–53
Iron
    autistic children status 84, 85
    complementary feeding timing effects on
      status 32, 33
    iron deficiency anemia effects in infancy on
      later cognition 49, 50

Leptin, birth weight and sex effects on levels in
  adolescents 3, 4

MC4, variants and body mass index 10, 11
Meal frequency, *see* Obesity
Metabolic syndrome
    childhood nutrition in adult risk
      prediction 17, 18
    probiotic studies in adolescents 19, 20
    vitamin D insufficiency 18, 19
Milk
    breastfeeding, *see* Breastfeeding
    low-fat milk studies of obesity in
      preschoolers 9, 10

Necrotizing enterocolitis (NEC),
  breastfeeding studies in extremely
  preterm infants 24, 25

Obesity, *see also* Leptin
    beverage sugar content studies
        body weight
            adolescents 5, 6
            children 4, 5
        cardiometabolic risk factors in
          adolescents 7, 8
        salt intake correlation 8, 9
    breakfast protein content studies in
      late-adolescent girls 14, 15
    carbohydrate modification in weight
      management in children 20–22
    complementary feeding
        food type and obesity risk 28
        timing studies 27, 28
    dietary pattern analysis in children and
      adolescents 13
    low-fat milk studies in preschoolers 9, 10
    meal frequency and body mass index
        genetic variants in adolescents 10, 11
        meta-analysis of studies in children and
          adolescents 11, 12
    probiotic studies in adolescents 19, 20
    vitamin D insufficiency 18, 19

Phosphatidylcholine, supplementation in
  pregnancy and cognition outcomes 46,
  47
Preterm infant
    breastfeeding studies
        extremely preterm infants 24, 25
        pasteurization effects on late-onset
          sepsis 25, 26
    colic, probiotic studies in breastfed
      infants 26, 27
Preterm infant, negative effects of rapid weight
  gain 98
Probiotics
    colic studies in breastfed infants 26, 27
    inflammation and metabolic syndrome
      studies in obese adolescents 19, 20
Protein, breakfast protein content studies in
  obese late-adolescent girls 14, 15

RESIST trial 15, 16

Salt intake, sugar beverage correlation 8, 9